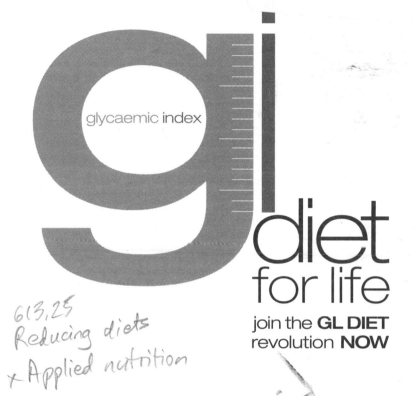

glycaemic index

gi diet for life

join the **GL DIET** revolution **NOW**

carolyn humphries

LONDON • NEW YORK • TORONTO • SYDNEY

foulsham

The Publishing House, Bennetts Close, Cippenham,
Slough, Berkshire SL1 5AP, England

Foulsham books are available from all good bookshops or direct from
www.foulsham.com

ISBN 0-572-03172-6

Copyright © 2006 W. Foulsham & Co. Ltd

Cover photograph by Terry Pastor

Photographs by Carol and Terry Pastor

A CIP record for this book is available from the British Library

With thanks for the following companies for providing the items for the photographs.

For herbs: Lavender and Stone, The Old School House, Upper Street, Stanstead, Sudbury,
Suffolk, CO10 9AU. Tel: 01384 753322. Website www.lavenderandstone.co.uk.

For all tiled backgrounds: Smith and Wareham Ltd. Tile Merchants, Unit 2 Autopark, Eastgate
Street, Bury St Edmunds, Suffolk, IP33 IYQ. Tel: 01284 704188/7.
Website: www.smithandwareham.co.uk.

For homeware and china: Crocks of Bungay, 9 Earsham Street, Bungay, Suffolk. Tel: 01986 892102.

For kitchenware and china: Marchants Cookware shop, 7 St Johns Street, Bury St Edmunds,
Suffolk, IP33 1SQ. Tel: 01284 705636.

For the preparation of the recipes: The Kitchen Machine / Cake mixer from the Kitchen Hardware
Professional Range by Morphy Richards. Website: www.morphy richards.co.uk.
Sharp Microwave oven: Sharp Electronics. Head Office: Sharp House, Thorpe Road,
Manchester, M40 5BE. Tel: 0161 205 2333. Website: www.sharp.co.uk.

Printed in Great Britain by Mackays of Chatham plc, Chatham, Kent

Contents

Introduction

This book isn't just for those of you who want a reducing diet. The GI diet makes great, healthy eating whether you want to lose weight or not. It positively encourages you to eat plenty of fresh fruit and vegetables (although you should go easy on the potatoes), lean meat, fish, poultry and low-fat dairy products, whole grains, nuts, seeds and pulses – in short, the sort of foods nutritionists recommend.

In the first part of the book I tell you how to shed excess pounds almost effortlessly, using the GI principle and an easy-to-follow diet plan. The second part is packed with innovative, delicious, tempting recipes for everyone, for every occasion and for every time of day. They are all carefully designed to keep your blood sugar levels fairly constant, so you won't have to face the problems of soaring highs and miserable lows. And they offer the perfect way to avoid feeling tired, listless and hungry and keep you feeling fresh and alert all day.

So, even if you don't want to 'diet', you can now enjoy meals that will keep you fit, healthy and bounding with energy.

A Simple Guide to the Glycaemic Index

In order to follow any diet, it is important to understand the principles on which it is based. This diet is based on the glycaemic index (GI) of foods, so let's take a look at what this means.

Your body converts carbohydrates (starches and sugars) into simple sugar (glucose) to be absorbed into the bloodstream for energy and this raises blood sugar levels – the level of sugar in your bloodstream. The glycaemic index of each food evaluates how much and how quickly this happens, compared (usually) with pure glucose, which is absorbed very rapidly. Glucose is given a rating of 100, whereas foods with no carbohydrates – such as meat, fish, poultry and cheese – are given a value of zero because they have little effect on blood sugar levels. Most foods that contain some carbohydrates are rated somewhere in between.

Foods that are slowly broken down into sugar for gradual release into the bloodstream will keep the level of your blood sugar – and so your energy – fairly constant. As a result, you are less likely to feel hungry and tired. These foods have a low GI rating (55 or less). Foods with a high GI value (70 or more), on the other hand, are converted and absorbed very rapidly. These quickly raise the blood sugar to a high level, which, in turn, will give you a quick burst of energy, then a slump, leaving you feeling tired, listless and hungry. There is also a secondary effect: when there's a surge in your blood sugar, your body, which can only use so much glucose in one go for energy, produces lots of insulin. This converts the sugar to fat to store it for later use when, maybe, it hasn't got enough for energy. Therefore, when you eat foods that raise your blood sugar quickly to a high level (a rapid glycaemic response), you start a vicious cycle: your body creates and stores fat, then your blood sugar levels plummet again and you feel sluggish and hungry. You immediately start looking for a snack to stave the off hunger pangs and give yourself a quick energy boost – and the cycle begins all over again.

So, in theory, if you want to lose weight, all you have to do is eat mostly foods with a low or medium GI, then you'll feel fuller for longer and so you should eat less. You won't need to keep snacking and you won't give your body the surges in blood sugar levels that cause the fat-making process.

Unfortunately, the reality isn't quite that simple. First and foremost, it is important for everyone to have a balanced diet, so some higher GI foods – like bread, pasta and rice – are a necessary part of it (although you should eat them in moderation). Also, some foods have a low GI value simply because they are very high in fibre, which inhibits the absorption of the sugar. And some foods have a low GI because their high fat or protein content makes them more difficult for the body to break them down but they are, in fact, high in calories. So despite their low GI, they won't help you lose weight. Good examples are full-cream milk, crisps (potato chips), chocolate and roasted, salted peanuts.

It is clear, then, that it's no good kidding yourself that every food with a low GI will help you to diet successfully – you need to identify those 'not-so-good' low GIs and eat them sparingly. Conversely, you should not assume that foods with a high GI will automatically make you fat. Some are actually very effective on a slimming diet: swede (rutabaga) and watermelon are good examples.

From this, you can see that using the glycaemic index is not an exact science. In addition to what I've already said, the rating itself can vary as a result of all sorts of influences and factors, such as:

- the quality of the produce (for instance, how ripe fruit is)
- how finely ground a grain is – the finer the grain, the quicker it can be absorbed so the higher its GI
- whether the food is already processed (instant mashed potato and quick-cook rice have a higher GI than their freshly prepared equivalents, because, being precooked, the starch is more quickly broken down and absorbed into the bloodstream)
- the amount of fat and protein mixed with the carbohydrates – this can slow down the absorption of glucose into the bloodstream, especially when several foods are cooked together

- the cooking method – frying, boiling and baking have different effects on the carbohydrates
- how long a food has been cooked – cooked starch is easier to digest so, for example, pasta cooked for 20 minutes will have a higher GI than if cooked for 8–10 minutes.

You will also find that GI databases vary and differ from each other in a number of ways. For example, I have used glucose as the benchmark but some databases use white bread as the measure instead. Check the value of white bread in any table you look at. White bread should be rated around 70 if glucose is used. If white bread is rated as100, then that has been used as the yardstick, which will make the values of other foods appear higher than the ones in this book. However, you will find that these variations are all in proportion to each other, so as long as you stick to one source (such as this book) you won't get confused.

How the index was discovered

Dr David Jenkins, a professor of nutrition in Canada, first devised the index in the early 1980s. It was designed for diabetics (whose bodies don't produce enough insulin, so cannot regulate their blood sugar levels naturally), to help them identify and avoid foods that have the greatest effect on blood sugar levels. He made some surprising discoveries. For example, he found that potatoes caused a rapid rise in levels, particularly when baked. This is entirely contrary to what nutritionists had always maintained. It had always been believed that complex carbohydrates – starchy foods, like rice, pasta, bread and potatoes – are broken down slowly and that the simple carbohydrates (sugars) are released into the bloodstream quickly. This was why it's always been thought that eating a chocolate bar would give you just a 'quick fix' of energy but then leave you feeling tired.

Soon it became clear that Jenkins's index would not only help people with diabetes, it could also help anyone who wanted to avoid storing body fat – in other words, anyone wanting to lose weight.

Note: Despite the medical background of the index, no one should go on this – or any other – diet without seeking a doctor's advice. If you are diabetic, it is even more important that you follow medical directions. However, you will find that the recipes in this book will give you a great base for a sustainable diet and lifestyle.

Glycaemic loading

The glycaemic index identifies which carbs are slow-release and which give a rapid response, but it does present one significant problem with using it to control your weight. The rating is meaningless unless it is related in some way to the quantity you eat. For example, jelly beans have a GI of 80 (high) but if you ate just one bean, it would hardly affect your blood sugar levels at all. If, on the other hand, you ate a whole packet, the response would obviously be very different! So, in order to get a true picture of what you are eating and how your body is reacting, you need to work out the effects of what you eat per portion, not just per food. This is called 'glycaemic loading'. Like the index itself, this cannot be an exact science, but it can act as a very good guide.

In this book, I've done the hard work for you: every recipe includes its glycaemic loading per serving and I have also included a chart that provides you with the glycaemic loading of an individual portion of many common foods. However, should you be interested, it is possible to work out the GL for any food yourself, using this simple formula:

$$\frac{\text{GI x carbs (in grams) per portion}}{100} = \text{GL}$$

So, for example, using the figures in my chart on pages 17–25, the glycaemic load of a ham sandwich made with 2 slices of wholemeal bread (15 g carbohydrates per slice) can be calculated as follows:

$$\frac{77 \times 30}{100} = 23.1$$

giving a round figure of 23.

(It must be said, however, that although the formula is simple, finding the GI and carb values of other foods may involve some time-consuming research!)

Using glycaemic loading to control your weight

By now you will have realised that just restricting your diet to low- and medium-GI foods is not a very efficient way to lose weight. Providing you pick the nutritionally sound ones and avoid the low GIs that you know won't help, like chocolate or crisps (potato chips), it would probably have some, albeit rather arbitrary, good effect. But in order to lose weight slightly more scientifically – and much more healthily – you need to turn your attention to the glycaemic loading figures – the GL.

In order to maintain a steady weight loss whilst supporting all your body's needs, you need to aim for a total daily glycaemic loading of around 70. This should come mainly from low-GI foods, with some medium and high ones too, to get a balanced diet. After an initial fairly rapid weight loss, caused by your body losing more water than actual body mass at first, you should then lose weight at around 450 g–1 kg/1–2 lb a week. This is quite gradual, but you shouldn't feel hungry or tired if you apply the plan correctly. Once you reach your target weight, you should be able to maintain it by working on a GL of up to 100 a day.

As I've said, this book makes this very simple for you. To calculate your total for each day, check the GL for each recipe serving or individual food you eat and add them all together. If you follow my recommendations, you shouldn't need snacks but, if you are a compulsive nibbler, make sure any in-between-meals additions come from the low-GI, low-calorie ideas on page 31.

Remember: it's no good just picking any random selection of foods that will add up to a total GL daily allowance of about 70. You must put together a balanced diet with a mixture of protein, carbohydrates, a little fat and lots of fibre, fruit and vegetables (see pages 11–12). Unless you are diabetic, there are times, too, when – surprisingly – you should eat food with a high GI, to raise your blood sugar levels quickly, such as after strenuous exercise. That's why sportsmen often have special isotonic drinks straight after they've trained or played and are recommended to eat more high-GI foods.

Quick tips for switching to a low-GI diet

- Eat wholegrain and seed breads.
- Eat lots of green, red and yellow fruit and vegetables.
- Cut down on potatoes, especially baked.
- Eat more legumes (dried peas, beans and lentils).
- Eat protein with high-GI foods to reduce their GI value.
- Eat lots of salads, dressed with oil and vinegar or lemon juice or French dressing.
- Choose unsweetened oat, barley or high-bran breakfast cereals.
- Avoid foods high in fat and/or added sugar, even if they have a low GI.

Maintaining a Healthy Lifestyle

I have talked about using the GI principle to control your weight. In this chapter, we examine the importance of other factors in maintaining a healthy body.

Remember that before you make any drastic changes to your diet, you should check with your doctor first. This is essential if you have any medical problem, such as diabetes.

A healthy diet

As I keep saying, in whatever way you choose to follow the GI principle, it is most important that you eat a well-balanced diet. You must eat foods from all the food groups below.

Proteins: These are used by the body for growth and repair and, when necessary, for energy. Best sources are fish, lean meat, poultry, dairy products, eggs and soya proteins – like tofu, Quorn (which is made from a fungus) and pulses (peas, beans and lentils).

Carbohydrates: There are two types of carbohydrates: 'complex' carbs include all the starchy foods like bread (all types), pasta, rice, cereals (including breakfast cereals) and starchy vegetables such as potatoes. 'Simple' carbohydrates are sugars and include those found naturally in foods – like fructose in fruit and lactose in milk – as well as refined sugars used in cakes, biscuits (cookies) and sweets (candies). The complex carbs and the natural sugars in milk, fruit etc., are usually considered the nutritionally 'good' foods and are used by the body solely for energy. However, when on a low-GI plan, some starchy foods are the foods that tend to have high GI values, so should be eaten in limited quantities. Refined sugars should always be avoided as they provide only 'empty' calories.

A note about fructose: you will find that fructose is used a lot in convenience foods and many GI diets use it as a sweetener as it has a lower GI than sucrose (ordinary sugar). I don't do this, because there is some concern that the body uses fructose differently from other sugars and can't easily convert it into energy, so it gets stored as fat if you have too much of it. In addition, it's not recommended as an alternative to ordinary sugar for diabetics. I therefore prefer to use a little honey instead. This is sweeter than any refined sugar, you don't need so much of it, and it has the added advantage that it helps boost the supply of antioxidants in your body so helps protect it against the effects of free radicals.

Vitamins and minerals: These are vital for general health and well-being. Many important vitamins and minerals are found in fruit and vegetables, both fresh and frozen, and canned in water or natural juice (with no added sugar and, ideally, no added salt). It is recommended that you eat at least five portions a day. Pure juice can constitute one portion a day only (however much you drink) but eating the items, rather than drinking their juice, is much more beneficial.

Fats: These are used for warmth and to keep your body functioning properly. They can also be converted into energy if enough sugar is not present, but this is a slower process than converting carbohydrates. Essential fats (Omega 3 and Omega 6 fatty acids) are, as the name suggests, vital to good health. They support the function of the nervous system and keep nails, hair and skin healthy. They are found naturally in your diet, providing you eat plenty of the nutrients recommended in this list, so you don't need any more. Added fats are a different matter: they are loaded with calories, so keep them to a minimum – have just a scraping of olive or sunflower spread (or butter if you must!) on bread and use the least possible quantity of sunflower or olive oil in cooking. Avoid saturated animal fats: cut off meat fat, remove skin from chicken, have low-fat dairy products, like skimmed or semi-skimmed milk, not full-cream and so on). Don't kid yourselves that it's okay to eat loads of full-fat crisps (potato chips), chocolate or roasted salted peanuts just because you've found they have low GI values. They are loaded with calories due to their fat content and won't do you much good – particularly if you are trying to lose weight.

Fibre: This is vital for healthy body function. It also causes food to be digested more slowly so sugar is released more gradually into the bloodstream. Eat lots of dark green vegetables, raw nuts, seeds and whole grains.

Drinks: Make sure you drink plenty of water – from the tap, filtered or mineral or no-calorie flavoured waters, according to your preference. Ideally, have a glass every couple of hours. Some GI diets recommend that you avoid caffeine (contained in tea, coffee and cola) because it may trigger insulin production. I suggest that you drink weak, black (or with semi-skimmed or skimmed milk) tea or coffee or, if you prefer, choose caffeine-free varieties or have herb tea. You may also have no-carbohydrate (diet) soft drinks, carbohydrate-free clear soup and pure fruit juice. Do not drink so-called fruit juice 'drinks' or other soft drinks sweetened with sugar.

Alcohol doesn't have to be avoided completely (although it's a very good idea to cut it out) but it will quickly lower your blood sugar levels and should be limited greatly if you are trying to lose weight. Alcohol always contains calories, which are easily processed by the body and these will be burnt before any protein, carbohydrate or fat in your diet. Here are some useful tips to follow:

- Have at least two alcohol-free days a week.
- Drink no more than 14 units a week for a woman,
  21 units a week for a man.
- Choose dry wine or spirits.
- Avoid beers and stout and all sweet alcoholic drinks, such as sweet cider, dessert wines, fortified wines (sherry, port and red vermouth) and liqueurs, as they contain significant amounts of carbohydrates.

- Always have no-calorie mixers or water with spirits.
- Drink plenty of water before and after drinking alcohol. Also, ideally, eat foods high in protein when drinking alcohol.
- Do not store up units and then binge-drink.

Energise with exercise

It is very important that you take regular exercise if you want to keep fit and healthy. That doesn't have to mean going to the gym and putting yourself through a weekly session of hell. Just 30 minutes a day of moderate exercise is much better.

There are lots of ways you can incorporate more exercise into your everyday life. Have a brisk walk at lunchtime, play an active sport, go for a swim, do some gardening or, if really necessary, go up and down stairs until your legs ache! Park at the furthest end of the car park from where you intend to go (instead of finding the bay right by the entrance). If you travel by bus, get off a stop early and walk the rest of the way. If you travel by train and the station is not very far away, leave the car at home and walk to the station instead. Get up a bit earlier and walk the children to school. Drag your bike out of the shed and cycle to the shops or work. Take the kids out on their bikes too. Take the stairs instead of the lift or escalator in shops or other institutions.

Obviously, doing sets of exercises, such as 'sit-ups', side bends, star jumps, leg stretches and so on, is also good (but check with your doctor if you are very over-weight or if you have any sort of illness). Incorporate them into your daily routine, say, before your shower in the morning or just before you go to bed at night, making them as much as part of it as brushing your teeth. That way you might just stick to them. Trying to fit them in whenever you can grab a few minutes simply won't work – once the first flush of enthusiasm has worn off you will find you keep 'forgetting'!

Posture

The way you hold yourself is also important. Stand in front of the mirror sideways and look closely. Are your shoulders hunched and rounded? Is your stomach sagging? Is your bottom sticking out? Now imagine you have a piece of string attached to the top of your head, pulling you upwards. Let your neck lengthen, tucking your chin slightly in. Let your shoulders relax and imagine they are being pulled back gently from behind. Feel the blades slide down your back. Clench your buttocks slightly, pulling in your tummy gently. Breathe out, feeling your ribs shrinking down and inwards towards your waist. Look again: you should look taller and much more upright. That's the posture you are aiming for – even when you're sitting down. It's a fairly safe bet that, normally, you sit slumped in a chair with your spine curved, shoulders rounded and chest folded down towards your waist. That's what gives you pains in your shoulders, back and legs – especially if you sit at a desk for hours on end. Think tall and upright: it really does work.

At-a-glance Guide to GI & GL Values

The table in this chapter represents the basis of the recipes and menus suggested later in the book and also provides you with the opportunity to calculate your daily intake for yourself. Unfortunately, only about 5 per cent of foods have been tested thoroughly for their GI value. So, if you stuck to eating only those, you would have a seriously limited choice of foods. For the purposes of this list, therefore, I have used our knowledge of the foods and their nutritional values to give you estimated GI values of many similar foods so you can have a far wider range of foods to choose from. For instance, peaches have been tested but nectarines have not, but there is only 1 g carbohydrate difference and their other nutrients are very similar. Consequently, I feel it is fair to assume that their GI value will be almost, if not exactly, the same.

The GLs are calculated on the carbohydrates available in the portions listed. All GLs are rounded up or down to the nearest whole number to make daily calculations easier.

As I said before, do remember when choosing foods, a low GI (under 50) is not necessarily an indication that a food is good for you – and can in some cases be just the opposite – this applies particularly to foods with a high calorie count, such as chocolate, pizza, roasted, salted peanuts, etc.

Food	GI	Portion size	GL
All Bran, dry	42	25 g/1 oz/½ cup	5
All Bran, with skimmed or semi-skimmed milk	38	1 average serving	6
Almonds	10	25 g/1 oz/¼ cup	0
Apple	38	1 medium	5
Apple juice	41	1 tumbler	4
Apple rings, dried	29	1 ring	1
Apricots, canned in syrup	64	3 heaped tablespoons	10
Apricots, dried	31	1 apricot	1
Apricots, fresh	32	1 apricot	1
Arrowroot biscuits (cookies)	65	1 biscuit	5
Artichoke, canned	15	1 heart	0
Artichoke, globe	15	1 globe	0
Asparagus	15	6 thick or 10 thin spears	0
Aubergine (eggplant)	15	¼ medium fruit	0
Avocado	15	½ medium fruit	0
Bacon	0	1 rasher (slice)	0
Bagel	72	1 bagel	32
Baked beans, canned, drained	48	1 small (225 g/8 oz) can	15
Baked beans, reduced-sugar and -salt, canned, drained	43	1 small (225 g/8 oz) can	11
Bamboo shoots	15	¼ small (225 g/8 oz) can	0
Banana	52	1 medium fruit	12
Beansprouts	25	1 good handful	0
Beef	0	4 thin slices/1 steak	0
Beefburger, 100 per cent pure meat	0	1 burger	0
Beetroot (red beet), cooked	64	1 medium	4
Black beans, soaked and boiled	30	3 heaped tablespoons	5
Black-eyed beans, soaked and boiled	41	3 heaped tablespoons	8
Blueberry muffin	59	1 large muffin	22
Bread, multigrain	43	1 medium slice	9
Bread, white	70	1 medium slice	12
Bread, white, high-fibre	68	1 medium slice	9
Bread, wholemeal	77	1 medium slice	13
Bread and butter	59	1 medium slice	10

Food	GI	Portion size	GL
Bread roll, white	73	1 roll	12
Bread roll, multigrain	43	1 roll	10
Breadfruit	68	1 medium fruit	70
Broad (fava) beans	81	3 heaped tablespoons	5
Broccoli	15	4 medium florets	0
Bulgar (cracked wheat)	48	3 heaped tablespoons	14
Butter, margarine or other spread	0	1 small knob	0
Butter (lima) beans, canned, drained	36	3 heaped tablespoons	5
Butter beans, soaked and boiled	31	3 heaped tablespoons	6
Cabbage, all varieties, shredded	15	3 heaped tablespoons	0
Cannellini beans, canned, drained	39	½ large (425 g/15 oz) can	8
Carrot juice	43	1 small glass	3
Carrots, cooked	41	3 heaped tablespoons	2
Carrots, raw	16	1 large carrot	1
Cashew nuts, roasted, salted	22	1 small handful	1
Cassava, boiled	46	5 medium slices	15
Cauliflower	15	4 medium florets	0
Celeriac (celery root)	15	¼ small head	0
Celery	15	1 stick	0
Chapatti	66	1 chapatti	15
Cheese (all types)	0	1 small wedge	0
Cherries	22	10 cherries	2
Chicken	0	¼ small chicken	0
Chicken noodle soup, packet	1	2 ladles	0
Chicken nuggets	46	6 nuggets	5
Chick peas (garbanzos), canned	42	½ large (425 g/15 oz) can	8
Chick peas, soaked and boiled	28	3 heaped tablespoons	5
Chicory (Belgian endive)	0	1 head	0
Chinese egg noodles, cooked	33	1 slab	9
Chips (fries)	75	1 average serving	37
Chocolate, milk	49	1 standard bar	14
Chocolate, plain (semi-sweet)	43	1 standard bar	13
Chocolate, white	44	1 thin standard bar	5
Chocolate biscuit (cookie), filled or coated	52	1 biscuit	5
Coconut	10	¼ nut	1
Coconut milk	10	100 ml/3½ fl oz/scant ½ cup	0
Ciabatta bread	68	1 medium slice	18
Cod, in breadcrumbs	43	1 piece of fillet	4
Condensed milk, whole, sweetened	61	100 ml/3½ oz/scant ½ cup	34

Food	GI	Portion size	GL
Corn chips, salted	42	1 small bag	13
Corn cobs, baby	48	4 cobs	1
Corn on the cob	48	1 medium cob	8
Corned beef	0	1 thin slice	0
Cornflakes, dry	84	25 g/1 oz/½ cup	17
Cornflakes, with skimmed or semi-skimmed milk	59	1 average serving	16
Cornflour (cornstarch)	70	25 g/1 oz/2 tbsp	16
Courgette (zucchini)	15	1 large courgette	0
Couscous, cooked	65	3 heaped tablespoons	19
Cranberry juice drink, sweetened	56	1 tumbler	14
Cream, all types	0	1 tablespoon	0
Cream cracker	65	1 cracker	4
Crispbread, puffed	81	1 crispbread	1
Crispbread, rye	64	1 crispbread	4
Crispbread, wheat	55	1 crispbread	4
Crisps (potato chips)	54	1 small packet	6
Croissant, all-butter	67	1 croissant	13
Crumpet	69	1 crumpet	7
Crunchy cereal and fruit bar	65	1 bar	11
Cucumber	15	5 slices	0
Custard apple	54	1 fruit	13
Custard, canned or homemade	37	5 level tablespoons	5
Dates, dried	103	1 date	1
Dates, fresh	72	1 date	6
Dhal	11	3 heaped tablespoons	2
Digestive biscuits (graham crackers)	59	1 biscuit	6
Eggs	0	1 medium	0
English muffin	77	1 muffin	21
Fettuccine, boiled	46	1 average serving	20
Figs, dried	61	1 fig	3
Fish	0	1 fillet, steak or whole fish	0
Fish fingers	52	1 finger	2
Flageolets, canned, drained	45	½ large (425 g/15 oz) can	13
Flour, plain (all-purpose) white	70	25 g/1 oz/¼ cup	13
Flour, soya	34	25 g/1 oz/¼ cup	2

Food	GI	Portion size	GL
Flour, strong (bread) white	73	25 g/1 oz/¼ cup	14
Flour, wholemeal	76	25 g/1 oz/¼ cup	12
French stick	68	1 thick slice	19
Fromage frais, plain, low-fat	0	1 average serving	0
Fruit cocktail, in light syrup	55	3 heaped tablespoons	11
Gnocchi	68	1 average serving	9
Grapefruit, fresh	25	½ fruit	1
Grapefruit juice, unsweetened	48	1 small glass	5
Grapes, black	59	1 small bunch	9
Grapes, green	48	1 small bunch	7
Green beans (all kinds)	30	3 heaped tablespoons	1
Ham	0	1 slice	0
Hamburger bun	61	1 bun	15
Haricot (navy) beans, canned, drained	45	½ large (425 g/15 oz) can	8
Haricot beans, soaked and boiled	38	3 heaped tablespoons	6
Hazelnuts (filberts)	33	25 g/1 oz/¼ cup	0
Honey	55	1 tablespoon	7
Hummus	8	2 level tablespoons	1
Ice cream, dairy	61	1 scoop	7
Ice-cream, chocolate	37	1 scoop	4
Ice-cream, low-fat	50	1 scoop	4
Jam (conserve)	55	1 level tablespoon	5
Jelly beans	80	1 bean	2
Kiwi fruit	53	1 fruit	6
Lamb	0	2 thick slices/ 1 chop or steak	0
Leeks	15	1 medium leek	0
Lentil soup, canned	44	2 ladles	11
Lentils, green or brown, canned	52	½ large (425 g/15 oz) can	10
Lentils, green or brown, soaked and boiled	30	3 heaped tablespoons	5
Lentils, red, boiled	26	3 heaped tablespoons	5
Lettuce	15	A large handful	0

Food	GI	Portion size	GL
Linguine, boiled	55	1 average serving	28
Lychees, canned in syrup	79	3 heaped tablespoons	14
Macaroni, boiled	47	1 average serving	20
Macaroni cheese	64	1 average serving	29
Mangetout (snow peas)	15	3 heaped tablespoons	0
Mango	56	1 medium fruit	13
Marmalade	48	1 level tablespoon	5
Marmite	0	1 level teaspoon	0
Marrowfat peas, soaked and boiled	39	3 heaped tablespoons	7
Mayonnaise	0	1 level tablespoon	0
Melba toast	72	1 slice	8
Melon, cantaloupe	65	½ melon	8
Middle-eastern flat bread	86	1 bread	13
Milk, semi-skimmed	34	300 ml/½ pt/1¼ cups	5
Milk, skimmed	32	300 ml/½ pt/1¼ cups	5
Milk, whole	27	300 ml/½ pt/1¼ cups	4
Milk bread	63	1 medium slice	8
Minestrone soup, canned	39	2 ladles	6
Morning coffee biscuit (cookie)	79	1 biscuit	3
Muesli, dry	56	25 g/1 oz/¼ cup	9
Muesli, with skimmed or semi-skimmed milk	45	1 average serving	15
Multigrain bread	49	1 medium slice	9
Mushrooms	10	6 button or 2 large	0
Nectarine, fresh	42	1 medium fruit	5
Oatcakes, ready-made	57	1 oatcake	5
Oatmeal	51	25 g/1 oz/¼ cup	8
Oats, rolled	51	25 g/1 oz/¼ cup	9
Oil, all types	0	1 tablespoon	0
Olives	0	1 olive	0
Onion	15	1 onion	0
Onion, pickled (unsweetened)	10	1 onion	0
Orange	44	1 medium fruit	6
Orange juice, pure	52	1 small glass	4

Food	GI	Portion size	GL
Pak choi	15	1 head	0
Papaya	59	1 medium fruit	12
Parsnip	97	1 medium	21
Pasta shapes, boiled (average)	43	1 average serving	18
Pea soup, canned	46	2 ladles	14
Peach, fresh	42	1 medium fruit	5
Peaches, canned in heavy syrup	58	3 heaped tablespoons	8
Peaches, canned in natural juice	38	3 heaped tablespoons	4
Peanut butter	23	1 level tablespoon	0
Peanuts, roasted and salted	14	1 small handful	0
Pear	37	1 medium fruit	4
Pearl barley, boiled	25	3 heaped tablespoons	10
Pears, canned in light syrup	45	2 halves	10
Pears, canned in natural juice	44	2 halves	8
Peas, fresh or frozen	48	3 heaped tablespoons	5
Pecan nuts	10	25 g/1 oz/¼ cup	0
Peppers (bell)	15	1 medium pepper	0
Pineapple juice	46	1 small glass	6
Pineapple, fresh	66	1 medium slice	7
Pine nuts	10	25 g/1 oz/¼ cup	0
Pinto beans, canned, drained	45	½ large (425 g/15 oz) can	10
Pinto beans, soaked and boiled	39	3 heaped tablespoons	9
Pitta bread	57	1 small	10
Pizza, deep-pan	36	1 large slice	11
Pizza, thin-crust	30	1 large slice	7
Plum, fresh	39	1 large fruit	3
Polenta, cooked	69	1 average serving	31
Popcorn, unsweetened	55	1 small handful	7
Pork	0	1 chop or escalope or 2 thick slices	0
Porridge, instant, made with milk	66	1 average serving	20
Porridge, traditional rolled oats, made with water	51	1 average serving	15
Potato, baked in jacket	80	1 medium potato	38
Potato salad	63	3 heaped tablespoons	10
Potatoes, instant mashed, reconstituted	85	3 heaped tablespoons	15
Potatoes, mashed	77	3 heaped tablespoons	12
Potatoes, new, boiled	59	3 small potatoes	11
Potatoes, new, canned	65	3 small potatoes	10
Potatoes, old, boiled	63	2 medium pieces	11
Potatoes, roast	60	2 medium pieces	16

Food	GI	Portion size	GL
Pretzels	83	1 small handful	3
Prickly pear	10	1 medium fruit	1
Prunes	29	1 prune	1
Pumpernickel	41	1 medium slice	8
Pumpkin	80	3 heaped tablespoons	2
Raisin bread	54	1 medium slice	8
Raisins	54	1 small handful	5
Raspberries, fresh	38	3 heaped tablespoons	2
Ravioli, fresh, boiled	39	1 average serving	12
Red kidney beans, canned, drained	39	½ large (425 g/15 oz) can	8
Red kidney beans, soaked and boiled	28	3 heaped tablespoons	5
Rice, brown, boiled	55	1 average serving	20
Rice, jasmine, sticky	109	1 average serving	61
Rice, long-grain, white, boiled	56	1 average serving	22
Rice cakes	82	1 round cake	6
Rice (cellophane) noodles, cooked	59	1 average serving	34
Rich Tea biscuit (cookie)	55	1 biscuit	3
Risotto	69	1 average serving	36
Ritz-type crackers	55	1 cracker	1
Rocket	0	1 good handful	0
Rye bread	65	1 medium slice	7
Salami	0	1 slice	0
Sausage, pork	39	1 thick	2
Seafood	0	1 average serving	0
Shellfish	0	1 average serving	0
Shredded Wheat, dry	70	1 biscuit	10
Shredded Wheat, with skimmed or semi-skimmed milk	51	1 biscuit	11
Shortbread	64	1 finger	5
Soya beans, canned, drained	14	½ large (425 g/15 oz) can	1
Soya beans, soaked and boiled	18	3 heaped tablespoons	1
Soya milk, unsweetened	44	300 ml/½ pt/1¼ cups	1
Spaghetti, white, boiled	44	1 average serving	22
Spaghetti, wholemeal, boiled	37	1 average serving	20
Special K, dry	54	25 g/1 oz/½ cup	10
Special K, with skimmed or semi-skimmed milk	44	1 average serving	16

Food	GI	Portion size	GL
Spinach	15	3 heaped tablespoons	0
Split peas, soaked and boiled	32	3 heaped tablespoons	6
Sponge cake	63	1 average slice	16
Strawberries	40	3 heaped tablespoons	2
Stuffing mix (bread-based)	74	1 level tablespoon	2
Sugar (sucrose), all types	68	1 level teaspoon	3
Sultanas (golden raisins)	56	1 small handful	6
Sushi	52	1 piece	4
Swede (rutabaga)	72	3 heaped tablespoons	1
Sweet potato, boiled	54	4 medium pieces	11
Sweetcorn kernels, canned	55	3 heaped tablespoons	15
Taco shells	68	1 shell	4
Tofu	44	½ block	1
Tomato	15	1 medium tomato	0
Tomato juice	38	1 small glass	1
Tomato soup, canned	52	2 ladles	6
Tomatoes, canned	26	1 small (225 g/8 oz) can	1
Tortellini, cheese, boiled	50	1 average serving	20
Tortilla, corn	52	1 tortilla	7
Tortilla, wheat flour	30	1 tortilla	8
Vermicelli, boiled	35	1 average serving	18
Waffle, sweet	76	1 waffle	23
Walnuts	10	25 g/1 oz/¼ cup	0
Water biscuit (cracker)	78	1 biscuit	5
Watermelon	72	1 large wedge	10
Weetabix, dry	75	1 biscuit	10
Weetabix, with skimmed or semi-skimmed milk	54	1 biscuit	10
Wheat crackers	67	1 cracker	3
Wild rice, boiled	57	1 average serving	3
Wild rice mix, boiled	54	1 average serving	17

Food	GI	Portion size	GL
Yam, boiled	54	4 medium pieces	18
Yoghurt, flavoured, low-calorie (i.e. with artificial sweetener)	23	1 individual pot	1
Yoghurt, flavoured, low-fat	33	1 individual pot	7
Yoghurt, plain, low-fat	36	1 individual pot	3
Yoghurt drink, low-fat	38	1 tumbler	10

Your 7-day Low-GI/ Low-GL Diet Plan

This is a simple eating regime that you can follow without having to cook special foods. Each day's menus add up to a GL of around 70, which should guarantee you a gradual, sustainable weight loss. Of course, you must adhere to the quantities given in the plan – so don't be tempted to add in the odd extra slice of bread, potato, carton of yoghurt, etc. However, if no quantity of a particular food is listed in the daily menus – as in some of the vegetable accompaniments – you can eat as much as you like.

If you think you will be unable to stick to this regime, you can opt for a daily GL of up to 80 and still lose weight. So, if you find you are feeling peckish, choose snacks from the list on page 31 – but remember your total GL should be no more than 80 in any day.

You can use the 7-day plan exactly as it stands for your daily menus, or, if you prefer, you can mix and match the meals to make up your own days' plans, or choose any of the recipes in the book. Remember, however that your daily totals must add up to your chosen GL (70 or 80, depending on how quickly you wish to lose weight).

Once you have reached your target, increase your GL to between 90 and 100 a day, by adding snacks from the list on page 31 or complex carbohydrates – such as portions of rice or pasta – or fruit or vegetables with suitable GLs. If you start to gain weight, simply reduce your GL a little.

Day 1

Breakfast	1 small glass of pure orange juice
Total GL 22	Oat porridge, made with 40 g/1½ oz/⅓ cup oats
	Skimmed or semi-skimmed milk
	1 tsp clear honey

Lunch	1 avocado with prawns, dressed with 1 tbsp
Total GL 21	mayonnaise, and a mixed green salad
	1 slice of wholemeal bread and a scraping of reduced-fat spread
	1 flavoured low-fat yoghurt

Dinner	Grilled (broiled) pork chop
Total GL 27	Clear gravy, made with the meat juices and stock
	Apple sauce, made with ½ sweet apple, stewed
	3 small boiled new potatoes
	Runner beans
	3 heaped tbsp sliced carrots
	1 wheat or rye crispbread, a wedge of Cheddar cheese
	and a small bunch of green grapes

Day 2

Breakfast	½ grapefruit
Total GL 19	1 or 2 boiled eggs
	1 slice of wholemeal toast, a scraping of reduced-fat spread
	1 level tbsp jam (conserve)
	or marmalade (preferably reduced-sugar)

Lunch	1 bread roll, filled with ham, a tomato, cucumber, lettuce and a
Total GL 24	scraping of mustard and mayonnaise
	1 banana

Dinner	1 poached salmon steak
Total GL 26	A portion of wild rice mix (50 g/2 oz/¼ cup uncooked weight)
	Mangetout (snow peas)
	4 baby corn cobs
	½ cantaloupe melon with ground ginger

Day 3

Breakfast	1 small glass of pure orange juice
Total GL 20	1 Shredded Wheat, with skimmed or semi-skimmed milk
	1 small handful of raisins

Lunch	2 wheat tortilla wraps, with tuna fish, 1 tbsp mayonnaise,
Total GL 21	shredded lettuce, cucumber and sliced tomato and a few
	drops of Tabasco
	1 apple

Dinner	1 grilled (broiled) rump, sirloin or fillet steak
Total GL 27	Mushrooms
	1 grilled tomato
	3 heaped tbsp green peas
	3 small new potatoes
	1 slice of fresh pineapple
	1 scoop of low-fat ice-cream

Day 4

Breakfast	1 small glass of pure grapefruit juice
Total GL 20	2 rashers (slices) of grilled (broiled) bacon and 1 or 2 poached
	eggs
	1 slice of wholemeal toast, with a scraping of reduced-fat spread
	1 tsp honey

Lunch	2 slices of multigrain toast, topped with melted cheese
Total GL 23	OR a cheese sandwich
	1 tomato
	Pickled onions
	1 fresh peach

Dinner	Spaghetti bolognese, served with 75 g/3 oz (uncooked weight)
Total GL 27	spaghetti
	A large green salad
	Celery sticks with soft cheese
	1 apple

Day 5

Breakfast	1 small glass of pure orange juice
Total GL 20	50 g/2 oz/½ cup muesli, with skimmed or semi-skimmed milk
Lunch	1 hard-boiled (hard-cooked) egg, with 1 tbsp mayonnaise
Total GL 21	and salad
	1 bread roll, with a scraping of reduced-fat spread
	2 plums
	1 carton of plain low-fat yoghurt
Dinner	¼ roast chicken
Total GL 26	Clear gravy, made from meat juices and stock
	Broccoli
	3 heaped tbsp sliced carrots
	2 pieces of roast potato
	2 canned pear halves in natural juice with 1 tbsp low-fat
	crème fraîche

Day 6

Breakfast	1 small glass of pure orange juice
Total GL 18	Poached or grilled kipper
	1 tomato
	1 slice of wholemeal bread and a scraping of reduced-fat spread
Lunch	1 small can of baked beans (reduced-sugar and -salt) on
Total GL 29	wholemeal toast
	1 wedge of Camembert
	1 apple
Dinner	Chicken noodle soup
Total GL 23	Grilled (broiled) gammon steak
	1 poached egg
	3 heaped tbsp sweetcorn
	Creamed spinach
	1 carton of plain low-fat yoghurt
	A small handful of raisins

Day 7

Breakfast   1 small glass of pure orange juice
Total GL 23   1 Weetabix, with skimmed or semi-skimmed milk
1 rice cake, with a scraping of reduced-fat spread and Marmite
3 heaped tbsp sliced fresh strawberries

Lunch   3 crispy tacos, filled with grated cheese, shredded lettuce,
Total GL 25   tomato, cucumber, green (bell) pepper, chopped spring onion
(scallion), a dash of chilli sauce and a small spoonful of low-fat
crème fraîche
1 fresh mango

Dinner   1 grilled (broiled) lamb leg steak or chump chop
Total GL 22   1 tbsp redcurrant jelly (clear conserve)
3 baby new potatoes, boiled
Shredded spring (collard) greens
3 heaped tbsp French (green) beans
1 wedge of Gorgonzola
1 oatcake
Celery sticks

Low-GI, Low-calorie Snacks

You shouldn't feel hungry if you are eating low- and medium-GI foods but if you are a compulsive nibbler, don't pick a packet of crisps (potato chips), a bag of peanuts or a chocolate bar.

Here is a list of snacks that you can use to supplement your daily menus without breaking your GL loading limit. Go for any of the following:

Snack	GI	GL
• A finger of Edam cheese	GI 0	GL 0
• A small carton of low-fat cottage cheese	GI 0	GL 0
• Celery sticks	GI 15	GL 0
• A raw carrot	GI 16	GL 1
• A low-fat yoghurt	GI 23	GL 1
• 10 cherries	GI 22	GL 1
• A pear	GI 38	GL 4
• A peach	GI 42	GL 5
• 5 dried apricots	GI 31	GL 5
• An apple	GI 38	GL 5
• An orange	GI 44	GL 6
• A kiwifruit	GI 52	GL 6

Notes on the Recipes

- All ingredients are given in metric, imperial and American measures. Follow one set only in a recipe. American terms are given in brackets.
- The ingredients are listed in the order in which they are used.
- All spoon measures are level: 1 tsp = 5 ml; 1 tbsp = 15 ml.
- Eggs are medium unless otherwise stated.
- Wash, peel, core and seed, if necessary, fresh produce before use.
- Seasoning and the use of strongly flavoured ingredients such as garlic or chillies are very much a matter of personal taste. Taste the food as you cook and adjust to suit your own palate.
- Fresh herbs are great for garnishing and adding flavour. Keep pots of your favourite ones on the windowsill and water regularly. Jars of ready-prepared herbs, like coriander (cilantro) and lemon grass, and frozen ones – chopped parsley in particular – are also very useful. I use a mixture of fresh and dried in the recipes. Don't substitute dried for fresh when only fresh is called for (there is always a good reason why).
- Throughout the book, I have recommended the use of low-fat dairy products, including reduced-fat spread, although you can use ordinary butter or margarine if you prefer. Check that any fat used is suitable for cooking as well as spreading.
- All can and packet sizes are approximate. For example, if I call for a 400 g/14 oz/ large can of tomatoes and yours is a 397 g can – that's fine.
- Cooking times are approximate and should be used as a guide only. Always check food is piping hot and cooked through before serving.
- Always preheat the oven and cook on the shelf just above the centre unless otherwise stated. Fan ovens do not need preheating and the positioning is not so crucial.

Photograph opposite:
Sausage & Tomato
Breakfast Wrap (page 34)

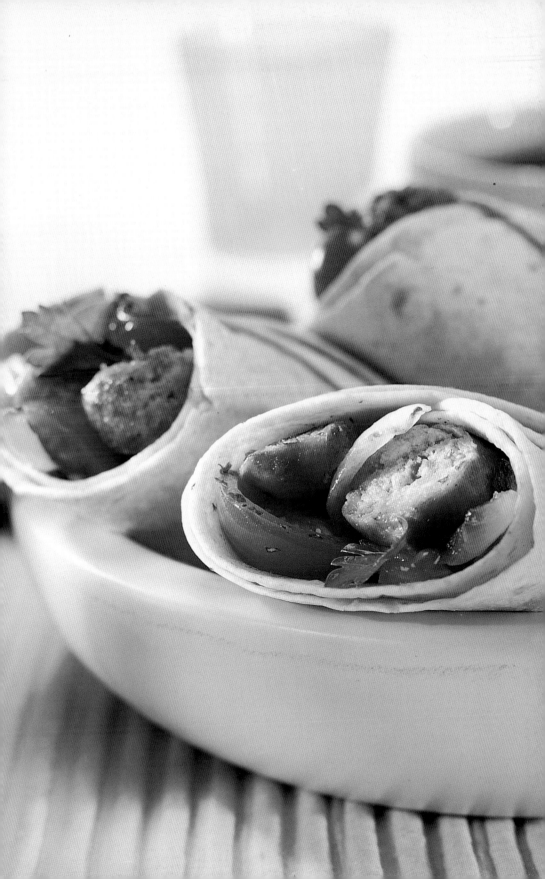

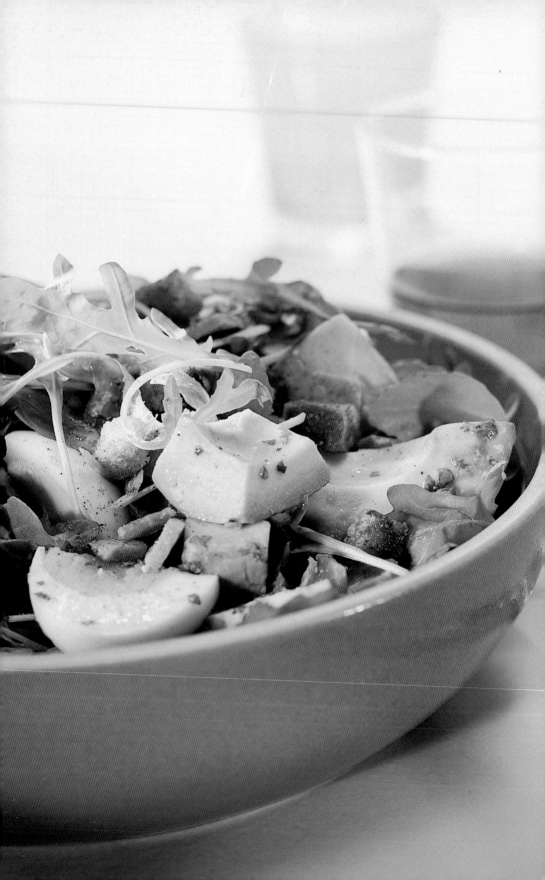

Breakfasts

Breakfast, we are frequently told, is the most important meal of the day – and it's true. The recipes in this section are designed to give you a boost that will start your day well and keep your energy levels high all morning, without making you feel bloated or listless.

Always have a small glass of pure orange or grapefruit juice (GL 4 or 5) as well as the accompaniments suggested in the recipes. You may also have tea or coffee – preferably decaffeinated (or at least not too strong) – with skimmed or semi-skimmed milk, if liked.

Photograph opposite:
Rocket, Avocado, Egg &
Bacon Salad (page 48)

Sausage & Tomato Breakfast Wrap

I particularly like spicy sausages in this for a truly Mexican flavour.
But any good, meaty bangers are fine. See photograph opposite page 32.

Serves 4

450 g/1 lb thick lean pork sausages
1 onion, chopped
12 cherry tomatoes, halved
10 ml/2 tsp Worcestershire sauce
Freshly ground black pepper
15 ml/1 tbsp chopped fresh parsley
4 wheat tortillas

1 Snip each sausage into six or seven small chunks with scissors.

2 Heat a non-stick frying pan, add the sausages and onion and fry, stirring, for 3–4 minutes until golden brown and cooked through.

3 Add the halved tomatoes and cook, stirring, for a further 2 minutes until softening.

4 Sprinkle the Worcestershire sauce over, add a good grinding of pepper and the parsley and toss gently.

5 Meanwhile, warm the tortillas briefly according to the packet directions.

6 Fold each tortilla into a cone shape and fill with the sausage mixture.

GL 12 per serving

Mushroom & Bacon Omelette Wedges

You can make a small individual omelette if eating alone – simply cook a quarter of the mixture in a small omelette pan and serve whole.

Serves 4

15 ml/1 tbsp olive oil
A small knob of reduced-fat spread
8 button mushrooms, sliced
2 spring onions (scallions), finely chopped
4 rashers (slices) of streaky bacon, rinded and diced
4 large eggs, beaten
Salt and freshly ground black pepper
Sprigs of fresh parsley, for garnishing
To serve:
4 slices of wholemeal toast and reduced-fat spread

1 Heat the oil and reduced-fat spread in a medium non-stick frying pan.

2 Add the mushrooms, spring onions and bacon and cook, stirring, for 2–3 minutes until golden.

3 Pour in the eggs and add a sprinkling of salt and pepper. Cook, lifting and stirring, until the mixture is just set.

4 Put a plate over the top of the pan, invert so the omelette tips out on to the plate, then slide back into the pan to cook the other side briefly.

5 Cut into wedges, slide on to warm plates, garnish with sprigs of parsley and serve with a slice of wholemeal toast, spread with just a scraping of reduced-fat spread, for each person.

GL 13 per serving

Smoked Haddock with Creamed Spinach on Toast

You can use other smoked fish for this recipe. I like to use the undyed variety but you could use the brighter yellow dyed fillets if you prefer.

Serves 4

350 g/12 oz undyed smoked haddock fillet
450 g/1 lb frozen chopped spinach
90 ml/6 tbsp low-fat crème fraîche
A good pinch of grated nutmeg
Salt and freshly ground black pepper
4 slices of wholemeal bread
A little reduced-fat spread
1 tomato, cut into 8 thin slices

1 Cut the fish into four equal portions. Remove the skin, if liked. Put the fish in a shallow pan. Cover with water. Bring to the boil, then reduce the heat, cover with a lid and poach gently for 5 minutes. Drain.

2 Meanwhile, cook the spinach in a separate pan without any added water for about 5 minutes until tender, stirring occasionally. Drain off the liquid, pressing the spinach against the sides of the pan to squeeze out any excess moisture.

3 Add the crème fraîche, nutmeg and a little salt and pepper and beat well. Heat through gently.

4 Toast the bread and add a scraping of reduced-fat spread to each slice. Place on warm plates.

5 Lay the fish on the toast and spoon the creamed spinach over. Garnish each with two slices of tomato and serve.

GL 13 per serving

Baked Sausage & Cheese-stuffed Mushrooms on Bagels

I like to make these up the night before, then just pop them in the oven first thing while I make an early-morning cup of tea!

Serves 4

225 g/8 oz pork sausagemeat
100 g/4 oz/½ cup low-fat soft cheese
15 ml/1 tbsp chopped fresh parsley
2.5 ml/½ tsp dried basil
Freshly ground black pepper
4 large open mushrooms
1 tomato, cut into 8 slices
2 bagels

1 Preheat the oven at 200°C/400°F/gas 6/fan oven 180°C.

2 Mash the sausagemeat with the cheese, parsley, basil and a good grinding of pepper.

3 Remove the stalks from the mushrooms, finely chop and mix into the sausage mixture. Peel the mushrooms.

4 Divide the sausage mixture into four portions and press a portion into each mushroom, covering the gills completely. Top each with two tomato slices.

5 Place in a baking tin and add 90 ml/6 tbsp water. Cover with foil.

6 Bake in the preheated oven for 10 minutes. Remove the foil and cook for a further 10 minutes until lightly browned on top and cooked through.

7 Meanwhile, split and toast the bagels. Place on plates. Top each bagel half with a stuffed mushroom. Spoon any remaining juices over and serve immediately.

GL 18 per serving

Ham, Egg & Avocado Pancakes

These low-GI/GL pancakes make an exciting change for breakfast, lunch or supper. Try them with some chopped green pepper instead of avocado.

Serves 4

25 g/1 oz/¼ cup wholemeal flour
Salt and freshly ground black pepper
5 ml/1 tsp dried mixed herbs
2 large eggs
150 ml/¼ pt/⅔ cup low-fat crème fraîche
50 g/2 oz cooked ham, diced
1 ripe avocado, halved, stoned (pitted), peeled and diced
2 tomatoes, seeded and diced
A little olive oil, for frying
4 slices of wholemeal bread
A little reduced-fat spread

1 Mix the flour, a pinch of salt and a good grinding of pepper in a bowl with the herbs. Break in the eggs, add the crème fraîche and beat until smooth. Stir in the ham, avocado and tomatoes.

2 Heat a little olive oil in a small frying pan. Spoon in a quarter of the egg mixture, spread out to coat the base of the pan and cook for about 3 minutes, tilting the pan from time to time to let the batter trickle round the edges and lightly golden underneath, until set. Flash under the grill to brown the top. Tip out of the pan on to a warm plate, cover with foil, and keep warm in the base of the grill (under the grill pan) while cooking the remaining pancakes in the same way.

3 Meanwhile, toast the bread, then add a scraping of reduced-fat spread to each slice and cut into triangles.

4 Arrange four triangles beside each pancake and serve straight away.

GL 13 per serving

Baked Bean & Bacon Scramble

If you don't want the bacon, omit it and melt a small knob of reduced-fat spread in the pan before adding the eggs and beans – it won't make any difference to the glycaemic loading.

Serves 2

2 rashers (slices) of back bacon, rinded and diced
2 large eggs, beaten
1 × 400 g/14 oz/large can of reduced-salt and -sugar baked beans in tomato sauce
Salt and freshly ground black pepper
2 slices of multigrain bread
A little reduced-fat spread
15 ml/1 tbsp chopped fresh parsley

1 Heat a non-stick saucepan. Add the bacon and dry-fry until the fat and juices run.

2 Add the beaten eggs and the beans and cook over a moderate heat, stirring all the time, until scrambled. Taste and season as necessary.

3 Meanwhile, toast the bread and add a scraping of reduced-fat spread. Place one slice on each of two warm plates. Pile the egg and bean mixture on top and top with the chopped parsley.

GL 20 per serving

Hot Strawberry Crumpets

These are gorgeous for breakfast or even for dessert or afternoon tea. You can experiment with other soft fruits, such as raspberries, blueberries or even hedgerow blackberries.

Serves 4

15 g/½ oz/1 tbsp reduced-fat spread
15 ml/1 tbsp clear honey
4 crumpets
100 g/4 oz/½ cup low-fat soft cheese
225 g/8 oz strawberries, hulled and sliced

1 Melt the reduced-fat spread and honey in a large frying pan. Add the crumpets and turn over in the mixture. Fry for 2 minutes on each side until lightly golden.

2 Slide out of the pan on to warm plates. Immediately, spread thickly with the cheese and top with a pile of sliced strawberries.

GL 10 per serving

Hot Oats with Raisins & Spiced Apple

You can make the porridge in a bowl in the microwave if you prefer. The cooking time will be the same. Stir two or three times during cooking.

Serves 4

175 g/6 oz/1½ cups porridge oats
300 ml/½ pt/1¼ cups skimmed or semi-skimmed milk
300 ml/½ pt/1¼ cups water
A pinch of salt
60 ml/4 tbsp raisins
15 g/½ oz/1 tbsp reduced-fat spread
15 ml/1 tbsp clear honey
2 green eating (dessert) apples, cored and sliced
5 ml/1 tsp mixed (apple-pie) spice

1 Mix the porridge, milk and water in a non-stick saucepan. Add the salt. Bring to the boil, stirring, reduce the heat and simmer for about 5 minutes, stirring occasionally, until thick and creamy. Stir in the raisins.

2 Meanwhile, melt the reduced-fat spread and honey in a frying pan. Add 60 ml/4 tbsp of cold water and bring to the boil, stirring. Add the apple slices and sprinkle with the spice. Cook for 2 minutes, turn the slices over and cook for a further 2 minutes until just tender and the liquid has evaporated.

3 Spoon the porridge into bowls. Top with the apple slices and serve.

GL 25 per serving

Warm Apricot & Yoghurt Crunch

To save time, you can cook the apricots the day before,
then reheat before serving.

Serves 4

225 g/8 oz/1⅓ cups ready-to-eat dried apricots
200 ml/7 fl oz/scant 1 cup water
1 cinnamon stick
500 ml/17 fl oz/2¼ cups plain low-fat yoghurt
1 crunchy cereal and fruit bar, crushed

1 Put the apricots and water in a saucepan with the cinnamon stick. Bring to the boil, reduce the heat, part-cover and simmer for 15 minutes or until tender and the liquid is syrupy and reduced.

2 Remove the cinnamon stick. Spoon the fruit and their juices into four dishes, top with the yoghurt, then sprinkle on the crushed cereal bar.

3 Serve straight away.

GL 16 per serving

Raisin Bread Bonanza

You can make this with other reduced-sugar jams and matching fruits, such as strawberry.

Serves 4

4 slices of raisin bread
A little reduced-fat spread
100 g/4 oz/½ cup low-fat soft cheese
60 ml/4 tbsp reduced-sugar black cherry jam (conserve)
10 cherries, halved and stoned (pitted)
40 g/1½ oz/¼ cup pecans, chopped

1 Toast the raisin bread and spread with just a scraping of reduced-fat spread.

2 Put one slice on each of four plates, buttered-sides up. Spread the cheese on top, then the jam.

3 Top with the cherries and then finally the nuts.

GL 14 per serving

Fruity Oat Breakfast Smoothie

Try this with a peach or pear instead of the apple. The GL will remain much the same.

Serves 1

1 banana
1 eating (dessert) apple, peeled, quartered and cored
15 ml/1 tbsp oat bran
200 ml/7 fl oz/scant 1 cup skimmed or semi-skimmed milk
A good pinch of ground cinnamon

1 Break the banana into several pieces and place in a blender goblet or food processor. Add the remaining ingredients.

2 Run the machine for several minutes until completely smooth.

3 Pour into a large glass and serve.

GL 23

Light Meals

These make great lunches or suppers. Many are suitable to be made into packed lunches for you to take to work – or to put in school lunch boxes – others are best left as treats for the weekends or rest days.

Don't be tempted to leave out the fruit or salad that I've included – they are vital to your healthy eating plan. I would suggest you also have a low-GI fruit, such as an apple, pear or peach afterwards or, perhaps, a low-fat yoghurt (but don't forget to add the GL to your total for the day).

Chilli Bean Tacos

If you are eating alone, make up the mixture and store half in a covered container in the fridge for the following day.

Serves 2

1 × 425 g/15 oz/large can of red kidney beans, drained
1 fresh green chilli, seeded and chopped
5 ml/1 tsp ground cumin
1.5 ml/¼ tsp dried oregano
1 green (bell) pepper, finely diced
2 tomatoes, chopped
5 cm/2 in piece of cucumber, chopped
4 crispy tacos
4 lettuce leaves
50 g/2 oz/½ cup grated Cheddar cheese

1 Drain the beans and place in a bowl. Mash with a fork, then stir in the chilli, cumin, oregano, pepper, tomatoes and cucumber.

2 When ready to eat, line the tacos with lettuce leaves, fill with the bean mixture and top with a little grated cheese.

GL 16 per serving

Hummus with Vegetable Dippers & Pitta Fingers

Warm the pitta breads if you can – they taste much better that way. If you are eating alone, store the second portion in a covered container in the fridge for the following day.

Serves 2

For the hummus:
1 × 425 g/15 oz/large can of chick peas (garbanzos), drained
1 garlic clove, crushed
15 ml/1 tbsp tahini (sesame paste)
30 ml/2 tbsp olive oil
Juice of 1 lemon
30 ml/2 tbsp hot water
2 large sprigs of coriander (cilantro)
Salt and freshly ground black pepper
For the dippers:
1 red (bell) pepper, cut into strips
5 cm/2 in piece of cucumber, cut into sticks
1 large carrot, cut into sticks
1 head of chicory (Belgian endive), separated into leaves
2 wholemeal pitta breads, cut into fingers

1 Put all the hummus ingredients except the salt and pepper in a blender or food processor and run the machine until smooth, stopping and scraping down the sides as necessary. Season to taste.

2 Spoon into small bowls and set each on a plate, surrounded with the vegetable dippers and fingers of pitta bread.

GL 14 per serving

Rocket, Avocado, Egg & Bacon Salad

Crisp, fresh, decadent – and one of my favourite lunches. If you're putting this in a lunchbox, pack the dressing and croûtons separately, then toss them together at the last minute. See photograph opposite page 33.

Serves 1

30 ml/2 tbsp olive oil
1 slice of wholemeal bread, cubed
2 rashers (slices) of lean back bacon, diced
1 small avocado
10 ml/2 tsp lemon juice
1 hard-boiled (hard-cooked) egg
A large handful of rocket
Salt and freshly ground black pepper
A few drops of Worcestershire sauce
A small handful of fresh parsley, chopped

1 Heat half the oil in a small frying pan. Add the bread cubes and fry, tossing, until lightly golden. Remove from the pan and drain on kitchen paper (paper towels).

2 Add the bacon to the pan and fry, stirring, until golden. Remove.

3 Halve, stone (pit) and peel the avocado and cut into slices. Add 1 tsp of the lemon juice and toss gently.

4 Shell the egg and cut into wedges.

5 Put the rocket in a serving bowl. Scatter the bread cubes, bacon, avocado and egg over.

6 Whisk the remaining oil with the remaining lemon juice, a sprinkling of salt and pepper and Worcestershire sauce to taste. Trickle over the salad, add the parsley, toss gently and serve.

GL13

Cauliflower Cheese Salad

Another winning combination of flavours and textures – this makes a delicious change from the more usual hot version. It's not worth making this salad for one, so share it with family or friends.

Serves 4

1 medium cauliflower, cut into small florets
1 bunch of spring onions (scallions), chopped
For the dressing:
100 g/4 oz/1 cup finely grated mature Cheddar cheese
30 ml/2 tbsp freshly grated Parmesan cheese
120 ml/4 fl oz/½ cup low-fat crème fraîche
120 ml/4 fl oz/½ cup low-calorie mayonnaise
Salt and freshly ground black pepper
Lettuce leaves
1 small handful of walnut halves, chopped
To serve:
8 rye crispbreads

1 Cook the cauliflower in boiling, lightly salted water for 3 minutes until almost tender but still with some 'bite'. Add the chopped spring onions for the last 30 seconds. Drain, then rinse with cold water and drain again.

2 Mix the cheeses with the crème fraîche and mayonnaise and season to taste. Add the cauliflower and spring onions and fold in gently,

3 Line four individual bowls with lettuce leaves and add the cauliflower mixture. Sprinkle with the nuts, then chill.

4 Serve with two rye crispbreads for each person.

GL 16 per serving

Spinach & Goats' Cheese Frittata

This is gorgeous served warm but is also good eaten cold in a packed lunch.

Serves 1

15 ml/1 tbsp olive oil
2 spring onions (scallions), chopped
100 g/4 oz frozen chopped spinach, thawed
1 × 75 g/3 oz round of goats' cheese, cut into small pieces
A good pinch of dried basil
4 cherry tomatoes, halved
2 eggs, beaten
Salt and freshly ground black pepper
To serve:
A soft multigrain bread roll with a scraping of reduced-fat spread

1 Heat the oil in a small frying pan. Add the spring onions and fry, stirring, for 1–2 minutes until softened and lightly golden.

2 Squeeze the spinach to remove excess water. Add to the pan and toss gently.

3 Scatter the cheese over the spinach with the basil and tomato halves.

4 Pour in the eggs and season with salt and pepper.

5 Cook, lifting and stirring the mixture gently, until the underside is set and golden and the top is almost set.

6 Place the pan under a preheated grill (broiler) until the top is lightly golden and just set.

7 Slide out of the pan and serve warm with the buttered roll. Alternatively, leave to cool, fold into quarters and place in the roll for easy transporting.

GL 10

Pasta Salad with Basil, Anchovies, Olives & Tomatoes

The lovely thing about jars of salted anchovies is that they keep in the fridge for absolutely ages, so you can make this any time!

Serves 1

4 salted anchovies from a jar
30 ml/2 tbsp skimmed or semi-skimmed milk
75 g/3 oz pasta shapes
1 garlic clove, halved
2 sun-dried tomatoes in olive oil, drained and chopped
6 black olives, stoned (pitted) and halved
4 baby plum tomatoes, halved
1 small green (bell) pepper, diced
15 ml/1 tbsp chopped fresh basil
15 ml/1 tbsp sun-dried tomato oil, from the jar
15 ml/1 tbsp olive oil
10 ml/2 tsp lemon juice
Salt and freshly ground black pepper
30 ml/2 tbsp grated Mozzarella cheese

1 Soak the anchovies in the milk for 15 minutes.

2 Meanwhile, cook the pasta according to the packet directions. Drain, rinse with cold water and drain again.

3 Rub round a mixing bowl with the cut sides of the garlic halves. Discard the garlic. Tip the pasta into the bowl.

4 Drain the anchovies and cut into pieces. Add to the pasta with the sun-dried tomatoes, olives, baby tomatoes, green pepper and basil.

5 Whisk the two oils with the lemon juice and a little salt and pepper. Pour over the salad and toss gently. Sprinkle with the Mozzarella and chill until ready to serve.

GL 18 per serving

Curried Chicken, Barley & Fresh Mango Salad

This is a great way to use up leftover chicken on Monday for a substantial but refreshing lunch. You can substitute turkey, if you prefer.

Serves 1

50 g/2 oz/¼ cup pearl barley
1 small mango, peeled and diced, discarding the stone (pit)
2.5 cml/1 in piece of cucumber, diced
2 spring onions (scallions), chopped
75 g/3 oz/¾ cup diced cooked chicken
For the dressing:
15 ml/1 tbsp low-fat crème fraîche
2.5 ml/½ tsp curry paste
15 ml/1 tbsp olive or sunflower oil
5 ml/1 tsp lemon juice
A small handful of chopped fresh coriander (cilantro)
Salt and freshly ground black pepper

1 Cook the barley in plenty of boiling, lightly salted water for about 30 minutes until just tender. Drain, rise with cold water and drain again. Tip into a bowl.

2 Add the mango, cucumber, spring onions and chicken. Toss gently.

3 Blend all the dressing ingredients together, reserving about half of the coriander, and season to taste. Pour over the salad and toss gently.

4 Pile on to a plate or, if taking for a packed lunch, tip into a container with a sealable lid. Sprinkle with the remaining coriander.

GL 23 per serving

Green Minestrone with Pesto

It's not worth making soup for one so if you are eating alone, you can always store any remainder in the fridge or, better still, freeze it in portions for use over the next few weeks.

Serves 4

15 ml/1 tbsp olive oil
1 onion, chopped
1 leek, chopped
1 courgette (zucchini), chopped
1 litre/1¾ pts/4¼ cups vegetable stock, made with 2 stock cubes
¼ small green cabbage, shredded
1 × 400 g/14 oz/large can of flageolets, drained
1 bay leaf
2.5 ml/½ tsp dried basil
30 ml/2 tbsp green pesto
Salt and freshly ground black pepper
Freshly grated Parmesan cheese, for garnishing
To serve:
4 multigrain bread rolls

1 Heat the oil in a large saucepan. Add the onion and leek and cook fairly gently, stirring, for 2 minutes until softened but not browned.

2 Add all the remaining ingredients except the pesto, salt and pepper and Parmesan. Bring to the boil, then reduce the heat, part-cover and simmer for 15 minutes. Remove the bay leaf, stir in the pesto and season to taste.

3 Ladle into warm bowls, sprinkle with Parmesan and serve each portion with a multigrain roll.

GL 16 per serving

Pancetta & Wild Mushroom Quiche

You can use diced streaky bacon and chopped button mushrooms, if you prefer.

Serves 4

4 slices of wholemeal bread from a large loaf, crusts removed
A little reduced-fat spread
50 g/2 oz diced pancetta
50 g/2 oz wild mushrooms, chopped
2.5 ml/½ tsp dried oregano
40 g/1½ oz/⅓ cup grated Cheddar cheese
1 egg
75 ml/5 tbsp skimmed or semi-skimmed milk
Salt and freshly ground black pepper
15 ml/1 tbsp chopped fresh parsley
To serve:
Cherry tomatoes and diced cucumber

1 Preheat the oven at 190°C/375°F/gas 5/fan oven 170°C.

2 Roll the bread slices with a rolling pin to flatten, then spread with just a scraping of reduced-fat spread. Place one slice, buttered-side out, in each of four individual flan dishes (pie pans) or ramekin dishes (custard cups), lined with non-stick baking parchment.

3 Bake the cases in the oven for 20 minutes until golden.

4 Meanwhile, cook the pancetta in a small saucepan until the fat runs, stirring. Add the mushrooms and cook, stirring, for 2 minutes to soften. Tip into the bread cases. Sprinkle with the oregano and cheese.

5 Beat the egg and milk together with a little salt and pepper. Pour into the flans. Sprinkle with the parsley and bake in the oven for about 25 minutes until set and golden. Leave to cool. Remove from the dishes and discard the paper.

6 Serve warm or cold with cherry tomatoes and diced cucumber.

GL 13 per serving

Celeriac, Barley & Cheese Potage

This warming soup has a rich and delicious flavour,
which is ideal for colder days.

Serves 4

1 onion, finely chopped
1 garlic clove, crushed
A small knob of reduced-fat spread
1 small celeriac, grated
100 g/4 oz/generous ½ cup pearl barley
1.2 litres/2 pts/5 cups vegetable stock, made with 2 stock cubes
1 bouquet garni sachet
Salt and freshly ground black pepper
30 ml/2 tbsp chopped fresh parsley, plus a little extra for garnishing
60 ml/4 tbsp low-fat crème fraîche
100 g/4 oz/1 cup grated Cheddar cheese

1 Cook the onion and garlic gently in the reduced-fat spread for 2 minutes, stirring, until softened but not browned.

2 Add all the remaining ingredients except the parsley, crème fraîche and cheese. Bring to the boil, then reduce the heat, part-cover and simmer for 40 minutes until the barley is really tender. Discard the bouquet garni, stir in the parsley, crème fraîche and cheese. Taste and re-season, if necessary.

3 Ladle the soup into warm bowls and sprinkle with a little extra chopped parsley.

GL 5 per serving

Tomato, White Bean & Fennel Soup with Olive Rouille

The olive rouille adds a delicious, rich touch to the soup but also makes a fabulous nil-GI dip with crudités. But, if you have lots of weight to lose, omit it and add a sprinkling of grated Parmesan instead.

Serves 4

15 ml/1 tbsp olive oil
1 onion, finely chopped
1 garlic clove, crushed
1 head of fennel, finely chopped, reserving the green fronds
1 × 400 g/14 oz/large can of chopped tomatoes
1 × 425 g/15 oz/large can of haricot (navy) beans, drained
600 ml/1 pt/2½ cups chicken or vegetable stock,
made with 1 stock cube
90 ml/6 tbsp dry white wine
15 ml/1 tbsp tomato purée (paste)
2.5 ml/½ tsp clear honey
2.5 ml/½ tsp dried mixed herbs
Salt and freshly ground black pepper
For the rouille:
30 ml/2 tbsp low-calorie mayonnaise
30 ml/2 tbsp low-fat crème fraîche
10 ml/2 tsp olive oil
1 garlic clove, crushed
8 stoned (pitted) green olives, chopped
2.5 ml/½ tsp lemon juice
To serve:
4 slices of melba toast

1 Heat the oil in a large saucepan. Add the onion, garlic and fennel and cook, stirring over a fairly gentle heat, for 2 minutes until softened but not browned.

2 Add all the remaining ingredients except the salt and pepper. Bring to the boil, then reduce the heat, part-cover and simmer for 25 minutes until really tender. Season to taste.

3 Make the rouille. Beat the mayonnaise, crème fraîche and oil together until glossy, then beat in the garlic, olives and lemon juice. Season to taste.

4 Ladle the soup into bowls and serve with the rouille and one slice of melba toast per serving.

GL 11 per serving

Tomato, Prosciutto & Mozzarella Wrap

This has all the flavour of the Mediterranean wrapped up in one easy-to-eat cone. You can add a few sliced black olives if you like.

Serves 2

2 wheat tortillas
4 slices of Parma (or similar) ham
1 tomato, chopped
1 × 125 g/4½ oz fresh Mozzarella cheese, drained and cut into small dice
6 fresh basil leaves, torn into small pieces
10 ml/2 tsp olive oil
Freshly ground black pepper

1 Put the tortillas on a board and lay the ham on top. Mix the chopped tomato with the cheese, basil and oil and season well with black pepper.

2 Fold the tortillas in half and half again to form flat cones. Open up and fill with the tomato and cheese mixture.

GL 8 per serving

Tuna & Sweetcorn Lettuce Rolls

If eating alone, store half the mixture in the fridge for use the following day.
Use the heart of the lettuce for a salad later.

Serves 2

1 × 185 g/6½ oz/small can of tuna, drained
1 × 200 g/7 oz/small can of sweetcorn, drained
30 ml/2 tbsp low-calorie mayonnaise
5 ml/1 tsp lemon juice
A few drops of Tabasco
Freshly ground black pepper
1 round lettuce
To serve:
Cherry tomatoes

1 Tip the tuna into a bowl and flake with a fork. Mix in the sweetcorn, mayonnaise, lemon juice, Tabasco and pepper to taste.

2 Separate the lettuce into leaves, including the large outer ones, but leave the tight heart intact. Rinse the leaves and pat dry on kitchen paper (paper towels).

3 Lay the eight largest leaves on a board. Lay a second leaf on top of each to reinforce it. Divide the mixture between the leaves, piling it in the centre towards the thick stalk.

4 Fold in the edges, then roll up firmly to form parcels – they should look a bit like spring rolls.

5 Chill until ready to serve with cherry tomatoes.

GL 15 per serving

Starters

For special occasions, it's lovely to have a starter before your main meal. When planning your meal, try to put together food combinations that complement each other by providing contrast and interest. Think about texture, colour and – obviously – taste, and remember not to overdo the quantities.

This section contains a whole selection that will provide you with plenty of ideas to suit every main course. What is more, they won't affect your blood sugar levels at all – the glycaemic loading is nil in every case, and they are low in calories to boot!

If you discover that your GL for the day is going to be very low, you can accompany your starter with a bread roll (GL 12), one thick or two thin slices of garlic bread (GL 19) or a piece of melba toast (GL 8).

Smoked Salmon with Lemon Mayonnaise

The lemon mayonnaise adds a refreshing twist to the smoked salmon. You could also experiment with low-fat soft cheese, moistened with a little milk, instead of the mayonnaise.

Serves 4

150 ml/¼ pt/⅔ cup low-calorie mayonnaise
Finely grated zest and juice of ½ lemon
Salt and freshly ground black pepper
30 ml/2 tbsp snipped fresh chives
8 thin slices of smoked salmon
A handful of whole chive stalks, for garnishing

1 Mix the mayonnaise with the lemon zest and juice. Season to taste with salt and pepper and stir in the chives. Chill until ready to serve.

2 Arrange the salmon on four plates. Put a dollop of lemon mayonnaise to one side and garnish each plate with a few chive stalks.

GL 0

Grilled Smoked Mackerel with Whipped Horseradish Relish

Smoked mackerel are often served cold but they are delicious hot, too. Grilling them in this way softens the fish and the relish offsets its richness.

Serves 4

75 ml/5 tbsp low-fat crème fraîche
30 ml/2 tbsp horseradish relish
1 egg white
4 smoked mackerel
15 ml/1 tbsp olive oil
2.5 ml/½ tsp dried mixed herbs
Wedges of lemon and sprigs of fresh parsley, for garnishing

1 Mix the crème fraîche with the horseradish. Whisk the egg white until stiff and fold into the crème fraîche mixture with a metal spoon. Chill until ready to serve.

2 Brush the mackerel with the oil and sprinkle with the herbs. Place on foil on a grill (broiler) rack and grill (broil) for 3 minutes until sizzling – do not overcook.

3 Transfer to warm plates, garnish with wedges of lemon and sprigs of parsley and serve with the whipped horseradish relish.

GL 0

Warm Spinach & Tomato Salad with Pine Nuts

If you can't get baby spinach, use wild rocket or a mixture of watercress and ordinary lettuce instead. See photograph opposite page 64.

Serves 4

60 ml/4 tbsp pine nuts
50 g/2 oz lardons (diced bacon)
50 g/2 oz baby spinach leaves, well-washed and drained
1 small red onion, finely chopped
12 cherry tomatoes, quartered
45 ml/3 tbsp olive oil
15 ml/1 tbsp oil from a jar of sun-dried tomatoes
15 ml/1 tbsp balsamic vinegar
2 sun-dried tomatoes in oil, drained and chopped
A good pinch of dried chilli flakes
Salt and freshly ground black pepper

1 Heat a non-stick frying pan. Add the pine nuts and toss until golden brown, then tip the nuts out of the pan on to a cold plate.

2 Add the lardons to the pan and cook, stirring, until golden and the fat has run. Remove from the pan with a draining spoon and drain on kitchen paper (paper towels).

3 Pile the spinach on to four small plates. Scatter the onion and tomatoes over, then add the pine nuts and lardons.

4 Add the oils and vinegar to the frying pan and bring to the boil, stirring. Add the sun-dried tomatoes and chilli flakes and season to taste.

5 Spoon over the salads and serve straight away.

GL 0

Grilled Camembert with Walnut & Tarragon Dressing

If you prefer, use four individual rounds of goats' cheese instead of the Camembert. You could also try using toasted pumpkin seeds with a dash of pumpkin oil in the dressing instead of walnuts and add a few halved cherry tomatoes to the salad.

Serves 4

50 g/2 oz/½ cup walnuts, chopped
60 ml/4 tbsp olive oil, plus extra for brushing
15 ml/1 tbsp walnut oil
30 ml/2 tbsp balsamic vinegar
2.5 ml/½ tsp dried tarragon
Salt and freshly ground black pepper
4 handfuls of mixed leaf salad
1 × 250 g/9 oz Camembert cheese, cut into quarters

1 Whisk the walnuts with the oils, vinegar, tarragon and a pinch of salt and pepper and leave to stand until ready to serve.

2 Put the salad on four small plates and spoon the dressing over.

3 Place the pieces of Camembert on oiled foil on a grill (broiler) rack. Brush with a little oil. Grill (broil) for 2 minutes until just beginning to melt. Quickly put on top of the salads and serve straight away.

GL 0

*Photograph opposite:
Warm Spinach & Tomato
Salad with Pine Nuts (page 63)*

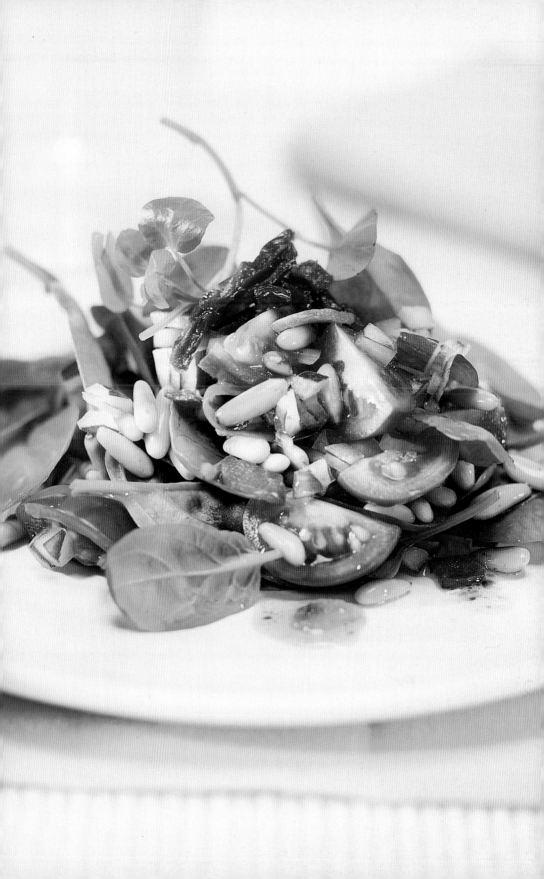

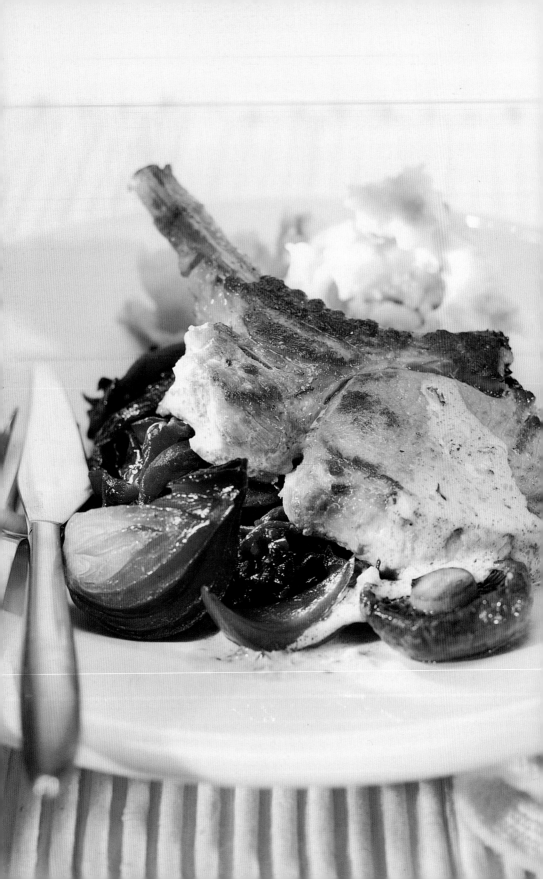

Chilled Mushrooms in Wine with Garlic & Tomatoes

This is also delicious hot, served with wild rice mix, for a vegetarian main course for 2–3 people. However, the flavours have more time to develop when it is chilled.

Serves 4–6

60 ml/4 tbsp olive oil
1 onion, finely chopped
1 large garlic clove, crushed
2 beefsteak tomatoes, skinned and chopped
300 ml/½ pt/1¼ cups dry white wine
1 bouquet garni sachet
400 g/14 oz baby button mushrooms, trimmed but left whole
Salt and freshly ground black pepper
Lettuce leaves and 30 ml/2 tbsp chopped fresh parsley, for garnishing

1 Heat the oil in a large saucepan. Add the onion and garlic and cook gently, stirring, for 3 minutes until softened but not browned.

2 Add the remaining ingredients. Bring to the boil, then reduce the heat and simmer fairly gently for about 15 minutes, stirring once or twice until the mushrooms are cooked and bathed in a rich sauce.

3 Remove from the heat and turn into a plastic container with a lid, cover and leave until completely cold. Chill for several hours or overnight.

4 When ready to serve, discard the bouquet garni, taste and re-season, if necessary.

5 Line four shallow dishes with lettuce leaves. Spoon mushrooms into the bowls and garnish with the chopped parsley.

GL 0

Photograph opposite:
Creamy Mushroom-topped Pork Chops
with Red Cabbage (pages 78–9)

Chorizo with Avocado & Fresh Basil Salsa

You could use salami, mortadella or any prosciutto instead of the chorizo for a change.

Serves 4

1 ripe avocado
1 celery stick, chopped
2 tomatoes, diced
5 cm/2 in piece of cucumber, diced
2 spring onions (scallions), chopped
8 large fresh basil leaves, torn
Salt and freshly ground black pepper
30 ml/2 tbsp olive oil
10 ml/2 tsp red wine vinegar
12–16 slices of thinly sliced chorizo

1 Halve, stone (pit), peel and dice the avocado. Put in a bowl and mix with the celery, tomatoes, cucumber, spring onions and basil.

2 Season lightly and toss in the oil and red wine vinegar.

3 Arrange the slices of chorizo attractively on four plates and add a spoonful of the salsa to each one.

GL 0

Parma Ham with Artichokes & Olives

Parma ham is so often accompanied by melon or other fresh fruit but there are plenty of other delicious ways to serve it. Here the artichokes and olives make a lovely savoury Mediterranean salsa.

Serves 4

1 × 400 g/14 oz/large can of artichoke hearts, drained and quartered
12 stoned (pitted) black olives, halved
1 green (bell) pepper, diced
45 ml/3 tbsp olive oil
10 ml/2 tsp lemon juice
Salt and freshly ground black pepper
5 ml/1 tsp finely chopped fresh rosemary
8 slices of Parma (or similar) ham
Tiny sprigs of fresh rosemary, for garnishing

1 Mix the artichoke hearts with the olives and green pepper.

2 Trickle the oil and lemon juice over. Add a sprinkling of salt, a good grinding of pepper and the rosemary. Toss well and chill for 30 minutes to allow the flavours to develop.

3 Curl the ham attractively and arrange on small plates with a pile of the artichoke mixture to one side and add a tiny sprig of rosemary to garnish each one.

GL 0

Griddled Asparagus with Quails' Eggs & Parmesan

If you have an electric health grill, cook the asparagus in that for just 2–3 minutes in total.

Serves 4

24 thin asparagus spears (about 450 g/1 lb)
60 ml/4 tbsp olive oil
8 quails' eggs
About 40 g/1½ oz/⅓ cup fresh shavings of Parmesan cheese
A sprinkling of coarse sea salt

1 Trim about 2.5 cm/1 in off the ends of the asparagus spears. Toss the spears in half the oil.

2 Heat a large griddle pan. Add the asparagus and cook for about 4 minutes on each side until the spears are just tender and their bright green colour is striped with griddle marks.

3 Meanwhile, put the eggs in a pan with just enough water to cover. Bring to the boil and boil for 1 minute only before plunging them into cold water to prevent further cooking. Gently shell the eggs, taking care not to break them as they will be soft in the centre.

4 Transfer the asparagus to four warm plates and drizzle with the remaining olive oil. Put two eggs on top of each serving and carefully cut them in half so the yolks run.

5 Sprinkle with shavings of Parmesan and a few crystals of coarse sea salt and serve straight away.

GL 0

King Prawns
with Chilli & Garlic

Prawns and garlic are a tried and trusted old favourite combination.
Here the addition of chilli gives them a real kick!

Serves 4

400 g/14 oz raw tiger prawns (jumbo shrimp), thawed if frozen,
shelled but with the tails left on
60 ml/4 tbsp olive oil
25 g/1 oz/2 tbsp reduced-fat spread
1 fresh green chilli, seeded and chopped
1 large garlic clove, finely chopped
Salt and freshly ground black pepper
30 ml/2 tbsp chopped fresh parsley
Wedges of lemon, for garnishing

1 Pat the prawns dry on kitchen paper (paper towels).

2 Heat the oil and reduced-fat spread in a large pan. Add the prawns and fry, stirring and turning, for about 2–3 minutes, until pink all over.

3 Add the chilli and garlic and season lightly with salt and pepper.

4 Transfer the prawns and their juices to warm plates or shallow dishes. Sprinkle with chopped parsley and serve garnished with wedges of lemon.

GL 0

Aubergines with Baby Plum Tomatoes & Mozzarella

This is another version of an old Italian favourite. You just can't beat the flavour combination!

Serves 4

1 aubergine (eggplant), trimmed and cut into 4 slices lengthways
Olive oil
2 spring onions (scallions), finely chopped
225 g/8 oz baby plum tomatoes, halved
15 ml/1 tbsp chopped fresh basil
Salt and freshly ground black pepper
100 g/4 oz/1 cup grated Mozzarella cheese
Small sprigs of fresh basil, for garnishing

1 Brush the slices of aubergine on both sides with oil.

2 Heat a large, non-stick frying pan and fry the aubergine slices on both sides for about 3 minutes on each side until golden and tender.

3 Transfer to a sheet of oiled foil on the grill (broiler) rack.

4 Heat 30 ml/2 tbsp oil in the pan. Add the spring onions and fry for 2 minutes, stirring. Add the tomatoes and toss over the heat for 2–3 minutes until softening but still holding some shape. Stir in the basil and a sprinkling of salt and pepper.

5 Pile the tomatoes on top of the aubergine slices and top with the cheese. Flash under a hot grill until the cheese melts.

6 Transfer to warm plates, garnish with small sprigs of basil and serve,

GL 0

Meat & Poultry Main Meals

All meat and poultry have a GI value of zero but that doesn't mean you can go round eating gluttonous amounts of them! An average steak, a good-sized pork chop, two cutlets, one chicken or small duck breast, a quarter portion of a small chicken or 2–4 slices of roast meat (depending on thickness) – that's the sort of quantity you should be aiming for.

All the recipes in this section include accompaniments, so the GL rating given is for the complete meal. If you chose to eat without the serving suggestion, you can deduct the GL for it (to find that, see Accompaniments, starting on page 122). You can also add as many extra nil-GL vegetables or salads as you please.

Braised Beef with Red Onions & Green Peppercorns

This rich casserole makes a lovely change from beef in red wine. It is equally flavoursome and tender.

Serves 4

15 ml/1 tbsp olive oil
2 large red onions, sliced
2 large carrots, sliced
45 ml/3 tbsp wholemeal flour
Salt and freshly ground black pepper
700 g/1½ lb braising steak, trimmed and cut into large cubes
600 ml/1 pt/2½ cups beef stock, made with 1 stock cube
15 ml/1 tbsp balsamic vinegar
15 ml/1 tbsp tomato purée (paste)
10 ml/2 tsp pickled green peppercorns, drained
1 bay leaf
A little chopped fresh parsley, for garnishing
To serve:
Crushed Broad Beans with Herbs (see page 131)

1 Preheat the oven at 160°C/325°F/gas 3/fan oven 145°C.

2 Heat the oil in a flameproof casserole (Dutch oven). Add the onions and carrots and cook, stirring, for 2 minutes.

3 Season the flour with a little salt and pepper. Toss the steak in it, then add to the casserole and cook, stirring and turning until lightly browned all over. Remove the casserole from the heat and gradually stir in the stock. Return to the heat and bring to the boil, stirring.

4 Stir in the vinegar, tomato purée, peppercorns and bay leaf. Cover and cook in the oven for 2–2½ hours until meltingly tender.

6 Stir the casserole, discard the bay leaf, taste and re-season, if necessary. Spoon the casserole on to warm plates with the crushed beans to one side. Garnish each plate with parsley and serve.

GL 9 per serving

Moroccan-style Lamb with Prunes

Lamb is often cooked with spices and fruit, such as apricots or raisins. I find prunes give added depth to the flavour and richness to the dish.

Serves 4

30 ml/2 tbsp olive oil
2 large onions, roughly chopped
2 garlic cloves, crushed
2 carrots, diced
450 g/1 lb lamb neck fillet, diced
5 ml/1 tsp paprika
5 ml/1 tsp ground cumin
5 ml/1 tsp ground cinnamon
150 ml/¼ pt/⅔ cup dry white wine
150 ml/¼ pt/⅔ cup lamb stock, made with 1 stock cube
15 ml/1 tbsp tomato purée (paste)
2 courgettes (zucchini), diced
12 ready-to-eat prunes, halved and stoned (pitted)
Salt and freshly ground black pepper
30 ml/2 tbsp chopped fresh coriander (cilantro), for garnishing
To serve:
Cumin Seed Couscous (see page 134) and a green salad

1 Heat the oil in a flameproof casserole (Dutch oven). Add the onions, garlic and carrots and fry, stirring, for 2 minutes.

2 Add the lamb and fry, stirring, until the cubes are browned.

3 Stir in the remaining ingredients. Bring to the boil, stirring. Cover tightly with a lid, reduce the heat and simmer very gently for 30 minutes. Taste and re-season, if necessary.

4 Garnish with the chopped coriander and serve with Cumin Seed Couscous and a green salad.

GL 22 per serving

Oriental Vegetable Steak Wraps with Egg & Mushroom Rice

You will need to choose thickish fillet steaks for this, so that you can slice each one horizontally into four thin steaks. If you have a friendly butcher, ask him for eight thin slices instead.

Serves 4

225 g/8 oz/1 cup wild rice mix
1 bunch of spring onions (scallions)
2 thick fillet steaks
45 ml/3 tbsp sunflower oil
5 cm/2 in piece of cucumber, cut into very thin strips
1 celery stick, cut into thin matchsticks
1 carrot, cut into thin matchsticks
45 ml/3 tbsp soy sauce, plus a little extra for sprinkling
50 g/2 oz button mushrooms, sliced
50 g/2 oz/½ cup frozen peas, thawed
1 egg, beaten
2.5 ml/½ tsp Chinese five-spice powder
30 ml/2 tbsp water
A good pinch of ground ginger

1 Cook the wild rice mix according to the packet directions in plenty of boiling, lightly salted water.

2 Meanwhile, trim and chop two of the spring onions. Cut the remainder into thirds, then slice into thin strips.

3 Lay each steak on a flat surface and cut horizontally into four slices. Place the slices one at a time in a plastic bag and beat with a rolling pin or meat mallet until very thin.

4 Heat 15 ml/1 tbsp of the oil in a frying pan or wok and stir-fry the prepared vegetable sticks for 2–3 minutes until softened but still with some 'bite'. Add 15 ml/1 tbsp of the soy sauce, toss well, then tip on to a plate.

5 Lay the pieces of steak on a board. Divide the vegetables amongst them, then fold the steak pieces over the vegetables and secure with cocktail sticks (toothpicks).

6 Drain the rice. Heat 15 ml/1 tbsp of the remaining oil in the saucepan. Add the mushrooms, peas and chopped spring onions and stir-fry for 2 minutes. Return the rice to the pan and toss so it is coated in the oil. Tilt the pan. Add the beaten egg and gradually stir it, drawing the scrambled egg into the rice. Season with the five-spice powder.

7 Heat the remaining oil in the vegetable frying pan. Add the steak parcels, laid on one side, and fry for 2–3 minutes turning once until browned and cooked through. Add the remaining soy sauce, water and ginger and allow to bubble for 30 seconds. Transfer the rice to warm plates and add the steak wraps and remove the cocktail sticks. Pour the juices over and serve straight away.

GL 17 per serving

Three-vegetable Moussaka

This colourful, tasty version of the Greek favourite has a very low GI so you need to add the garlic pittas to have a sensible GL – you must have some complex carbs every day to give you a balanced diet.

Serves 4

1 aubergine (eggplant), sliced
1 large courgette (zucchini), sliced
2 red (bell) peppers, cut into thick strips
350 g/12 oz minced (ground) lamb
1 onion, chopped
1 garlic clove, crushed
1 × 400 g/14 oz/large can of chopped tomatoes
15 ml/ tbsp tomato purée (paste)
5 ml/1 tsp ground cinnamon
5 ml/1 tsp dried oregano
5 ml/1 tsp clear honey
Salt and freshly ground black pepper
2 eggs
300 ml/½ pt/1¼ cups low-fat Greek yoghurt
75 g/3 oz/¾ cup grated Cheddar cheese
To serve:
Mixed Salad with Olives and Feta (see page 128)
and Garlic Pitta Fingers (see page 135)

1 Preheat the oven at 190°C/375°F/gas mark 5/fan oven 170°C.

2 Bring a large pan of water to the boil. Add the aubergine, courgette and peppers and boil for 3 minutes. Drain, rinse with cold water and drain thoroughly again.

3 Put the meat, onion and garlic in a saucepan and cook, stirring, for about 4 minutes until the meat is no longer pink and all the grains are separate.

4 Add the tomatoes, tomato purée, cinnamon, oregano and honey. Stir well and simmer gently for 10 minutes, stirring occasionally. Season to taste.

5 Layer the vegetables and meat in a shallow 1.75 litre/3 pt/7½ cup ovenproof dish, finishing with a layer of vegetables.

6 Beat the egg and yoghurt together with a pinch of salt and a good grinding of pepper. Stir in the cheese.

7 Spoon over the layer of vegetables. Bake in the preheated oven for about 40 minutes until the top is set and golden.

8 Leave to cool for about 10 minutes, then serve warm with the salad and pitta strips.

GL 22 per serving

Creamy Mushroom-topped Pork Chops with Red Cabbage

*Lean pork chops with a rich creamy mushroom topping served on a bed of
sweet and sour red cabbage served with fluffy celeriac and potato mash –
a perfect, warming winter dish. The dish is good served with button
mushrooms. See photograph opposite page 65.*

Serves 4

15 g/½ oz/1 tbsp reduced-fat spread
1 small red cabbage, shredded
1 red onion, halved and thinly sliced
50 g/2 oz/⅓ cup raisins
Salt and freshly ground black pepper
10 ml/2 tsp clear honey
60 ml/4 tbsp balsamic vinegar
30 ml/2 tbsp water
4 large pork chops
30 ml/2 tbsp olive oil
4 large flat mushrooms, peeled and finely chopped
2.5 ml/½ tsp dried oregano
150 ml/¼ pt/⅔ cup low-fat crème fraîche
30 ml/2 tbsp chopped fresh parsley
To serve:
Celeriac and Potato Mash (see page 124)

1 Melt the reduced-fat spread in a flameproof casserole dish (Dutch
   oven). Layer the cabbage, onion and raisins in the casserole,
   sprinkling each layer with a little salt and lots of pepper.

2 Mix the honey with the vinegar and water and pour over. Bring to the
   boil, cover tightly, then turn down the heat to very low and cook
   gently for about 40 minutes, stirring occasionally, until really tender.

3 Season the chops on both sides with salt and pepper. Heat the oil in a
   large frying pan and brown the chops quickly on both sides.

4 Turn down the heat to moderate and cook for 10 minutes until golden and cooked through, turning the chops once. Remove from the pan and keep warm.

5 Add the mushrooms and oregano to the juices in the pan and fry for 2 minutes, stirring. Add the crème fraîche and heat through but do not boil. Season to taste.

6 Transfer the red cabbage to warm plates, using a draining spoon to avoid any excess moisture. Put the chops on top of the cabbage and spoon the sauce over. Sprinkle with parsley and serve with the mash.

GL 14 per serving

Spinach-stuffed Pork Tenderloin with a Grainy Mustard Jus

The spinach stuffing has just a touch of citrus and some toasted pine nuts to add zing to the taste and texture, while the sauce adds richness and flavour.

Serves 4

2 small pork tenderloins, about 225 g/8 oz each
25 g/1 oz/¼ cup pine nuts
100 g/4 oz frozen chopped spinach, thawed
15 ml/1 tbsp olive oil, plus a little extra for greasing
1 garlic clove, crushed
30 ml/2 tbsp snipped fresh chives
Finely grated zest of 1 small lemon
Salt and freshly ground black pepper
150 ml/¼ pt/⅔ cup dry vermouth
15 ml/1 tbsp grainy mustard
150 ml/¼ pt/⅔ cup low-fat crème fraîche
To serve:
Carrot and White Bean Braise (see page 132)

1 Preheat the oven at 200°C/400°F/gas 6/fan oven 180°C.

2 Trim any sinews off the pork. Make a slit down the length of each, not quite right through, to form a pocket.

3 Heat a non-stick frying pan and dry-fry the pine nuts for about 3 minutes until golden, then tip out of the pan into a bowl prevent further cooking.

4 Squeeze the spinach thoroughly to remove excess moisture. Mix with the pine nuts and add the oil, garlic, chives, lemon zest and a little salt and pepper.

5 Pack the mixture into the pork tenderloins. Lightly oil a sheet of greaseproof (waxed) paper and wrap up the tenderloins tightly. Place in a roasting tin and roast in the oven for 30 minutes.

6 Remove from the oven. Carefully unwrap the pork at one end and pour most of the juices into a small saucepan. Rewrap the pork and keep warm.

7 Add the vermouth to the juices and boil rapidly for about 2 minutes until reduced by half. Stir in the mustard and crème fraîche. Heat through and season to taste.

8 Carve the pork into thick slices. Arrange on warm plates and pour a little of the jus over. Serve with the Carrot and White Bean Braise.

GL 5 per serving

Warm Pork, Rocket, Potato & Beetroot Salad

Another exciting combination for you to try. You could also use thin frying steaks or turkey steaks, beaten very flat.

Serves 4

12 baby new potatoes, scrubbed and halved
1 small pork tenderloin, about 225 g/8 oz, cut into 8–12 slices
15 ml/1 tbsp coarsely crushed black peppercorns
5 ml/1 tsp dried sage
4 small cooked beetroot (red beets), diced
12 cherry tomatoes, halved
A small bunch of fresh flat-leaf parsley
1 × 70 g/2½ oz/small packet of wild rocket
For the dressing:
60 ml/4 tbsp olive oil
1 spring onion (scallion), finely chopped
10 ml/2 tsp pickled capers, chopped
2.5 cm/1 in piece of cucumber, finely chopped
30 ml/2 tbsp balsamic vinegar
Salt and freshly ground black pepper
1 × 125 g/4½ oz/small carton of plain cottage cheese, for garnishing
A little olive oil, for cooking

1 Boil the potatoes in lightly salted water until tender. Drain.

2 Put the pork slices in a plastic bag and beat with a meat mallet or rolling pin to flatten. Mix the peppercorns with the sage and sprinkle on both sides of the meat slices.

3 Mix the potato, beetroot, tomatoes, parsley and rocket together. Pile on four plates. Whisk together all the dressing ingredients. Spoon over the salads and top with a spoonful of cottage cheese.

4 Heat a little olive oil in a large frying pan and fry the pork quickly for about 2 minutes on each side until golden and cooked through. Lay the pork on top of the salads and serve straight away.

GL 13 per serving

Chilli Chicken & Bamboo Shoot Stir-fry with Noodles

A spicy, quick stir-fry with loads of flavour and goodness. It makes a complete, filling meal and has a blissfully low GI and GL!

Serves 4

2 slabs of Chinese egg noodles
30 ml/2 tbsp sunflower oil
4 skinless chicken breasts, cut into strips
1 bunch of spring onions (scallions), cut into short lengths
1 fresh red or green chilli, seeded and chopped
1 green (bell) pepper
1 red pepper
1 small head of spring (collard) greens, finely shredded
1 garlic clove, crushed
10 cm/4 in piece of cucumber, cut into matchsticks
1 × 225 g/8 oz/small can of bamboo shoots, drained
30 ml/2 tbsp soy sauce
30 ml/2 tbsp dry sherry
2.5 ml/½ tsp ground ginger
5 ml/1 tsp clear honey
To serve:
Soy sauce

1 Put the noodles in a large bowl, cover with boiling water and leave to soak, stirring once or twice, while you cook the rest of the dish.

2 Heat the oil in a large frying pan or wok. Add the chicken and stir-fry for 2 minutes. Add the spring onions, chilli, peppers, spring greens and garlic and stir-fry for 3 minutes. Add the cucumber and bamboo shoots and stir-fry for 1 minute.

3 Add the remaining ingredients, including the drained noodles, and toss well for 1 minute.

4 Spoon into warm bowls and serve with extra soy sauce, if liked.

GL 6 per serving

Stuffed Tandoori-style Chicken

An exciting variation on ordinary tandoori chicken: the breasts are filled with a moist stuffing flavoured with coriander and garlic, then marinated and baked in the usual way. Use 1 heaped tablespoon of tandoori paste rather than the mixed spices, if you prefer.

Serves 4

For the stuffing:
25 g/1 oz/2 tbsp reduced-fat spread
50 g/2 oz/1 cup fresh wholemeal breadcrumbs
30 ml/2 tbsp chopped fresh coriander (cilantro)
30 ml/2 tbsp chopped fresh parsley
1 large garlic clove, crushed
Salt and freshly ground black pepper
4 skinless chicken breasts
150 ml/¼ pt/⅔ cup thick plain low-fat yoghurt
5 ml/1 tsp ground coriander
5 ml/1 tsp ground cumin
2.5 ml/½ tsp chilli powder
5 ml/1 tsp garam masala
10 ml/2 tsp paprika
2.5 ml/½ tsp garlic salt
For the raita:
¼ cucumber, grated
1 small garlic clove, crushed
150 ml/¼ pt/⅔ cup thick plain low-fat yoghurt
Wedges of lettuce, tomato and lemon, for garnishing
To serve:
Indian Spiced Potato, Celeriac and Onion (see page 125)

1 Preheat the oven at 190°C/375°F/gas 5/fan oven 170°C.

2 Melt the reduced-fat spread. Remove from the heat and add the breadcrumbs, herbs, garlic and a little salt and pepper.

3 Make a slit in the side of each chicken breast to form a pocket. Pack the stuffing inside and secure with a wooden cocktail stick (toothpick).

4 Mix the yoghurt with the spices and garlic salt in a shallow dish, large enough to take the chicken in a single layer. Add the chicken and turn it over to coat completely. Cover and chill for at least 3 hours.

5 Transfer the yoghurt-coated chicken to a baking tin, arranging the pieces in a single layer. Bake in the oven for 35 minutes.

6 Meanwhile make the raita. Squeeze the cucumber to remove excess liquid. Mix with the garlic and yoghurt and add a little seasoning. Chill until ready to serve.

7 Drain the chicken and transfer to warm plates. Remove the cocktail sticks. Garnish with the salad and lemon and serve with the raita and Indian Spiced Potato, Celeriac and Onion.

GL16 per serving

Sweet & Sour Chicken Breasts

This is a lovely variation on the more usual diced chicken in a sweet and sour sauce. It looks beautiful and tastes even better!

Serves 4

150 ml/¼ pt/⅔ cup pure pineapple juice
15 ml/1 tbsp cornflour (cornstarch)
15 ml/1 tbsp tomato purée (paste)
5 ml/1 tsp grated fresh root ginger
1 garlic clove, crushed
15 ml/1 tbsp soy sauce
4 skinless chicken breasts
For the garnish:
15 ml/1 tbsp sunflower oil
½ bunch of spring onions (scallions), halved and cut into thin strips
1 red (bell) pepper, cut into very thin strips
5 cm/2 in piece of cucumber, cut into very thin strips
1 carrot, cut into very thin matchsticks
To serve:
Sesame and Spring Onion Noodles (see page 127)

1 Blend the pineapple juice with the cornflour in a wok or large frying pan. Stir in the tomato purée, ginger, garlic and soy sauce. Bring to the boil, stirring.

2 Add the chicken breasts, tucking them down well in the sauce. Cover with a lid or foil, turn down the heat to low and simmer for 20 minutes, stirring once or twice.

3 When the chicken is nearly cooked, heat the oil in a separate pan. Add the vegetable strips and stir-fry for 1 minute only.

4 Check that the chicken is cooked through, then transfer to warm plates, spoon the sauce over and top with the stir-fried vegetables.

5 Serve with Sesame and Spring Onion Noodles.

GL 7 per serving

Peppered Liver with Red Wine Jus

This is quick, easy, elegant and extremely nutritious. Enjoy it midweek or as a special occasion meal. Make sure you don't overcook the liver.

Serves 4

350 g/12 oz lambs' liver
30 ml/2 tbsp plain (all-purpose) flour
30 ml/2 tbsp coarsely crushed black peppercorns
A pinch of salt
A small knob of reduced-fat spread
30 ml/2 tbsp olive oil
150 ml/¼ pt/⅔ cup red wine
90 ml/6 tbsp water
15 ml/1 tbsp tomato purée (paste)
2.5 ml/½ tsp clear honey
2.5 ml/½ tsp dried mixed herbs
30 ml/2 tbsp chopped fresh parsley, for garnishing
To serve:
Celeriac and Potato Mash (see page 124) and French (green) beans

1 Cut each piece of liver horizontally into two or three thinner slices, each about 5 mm/¼ in thick.

2 Mix the flour with the peppercorns and a pinch of salt. Dip the liver in the mixture on both sides to coat completely.

3 Heat the spread and oil in large frying pan. Cook the liver on one side until golden. Turn and cook just until droplets of juice appear on the surface. Remove from the pan immediately and keep warm.

4 Add the remaining ingredients to the pan and stir until bubbling and slightly thickened. Season to taste.

5 Transfer the liver to warm plates. Spoon the wine jus over and garnish with the parsley. Serve with Celeriac and Potato Mash and 3 heaped tablespoons of French beans per person.

GL 9 per serving

Pancetta-wrapped Kidney Kebabs with Devilled Sauce

Rich and delicious, kidneys are highly nutritious and very versatile. Here they are wrapped in pancetta to keep them moist, lightly grilled and served on a bed of saffron-flavoured barley risotto, dotted with tiny florets of broccoli.

Serves 4

For the kidneys:
12 lambs' kidneys
12 thin slices of pancetta
2 large courgettes (zucchini), each cut into 8 chunks
30 ml/2 tbsp olive oil
15 ml/1 tbsp lemon juice
2.5 ml/½ tsp dried mixed herbs
Salt and freshly ground black pepper
For the sauce:
15 ml/1 tbsp Dijon mustard
1.5 ml/¼ tsp chilli powder
30 ml/2 tbsp tomato purée (paste)
5 ml/1 tsp Worcestershire sauce
150 ml/¼ pt/⅔ cup apple juice
30 ml/2 tbsp chopped fresh parsley, for garnishing
To serve:
Saffron Barley and Broccoli Risotto (see page 129)

1 Cut the kidneys in half with scissors and snip out the central cores. Cut the pancetta slices in half and wrap one piece round each piece of kidney.

2 Bring a small pan of water to the boil and cook the courgette pieces for 2 minutes. Drain, rinse with cold water and drain again.

3 Thread three pieces of kidney and two pieces of courgette on to each of eight skewers.

4 Mix the oil with the lemon juice, herbs and a little salt and pepper and brush all over the kebabs.

5 Preheat the grill (broiler). Lay the kebabs on a sheet of foil on the grill rack. Grill (broil) for 6 minutes, brushing with any remaining oil mixture and turning once during cooking, until golden and just cooked through. Do not overcook.

6 Meanwhile, mix the sauce ingredients together in a small saucepan. Bring to the boil, stirring and simmer for 2 minutes.

7 Transfer the kebabs to warm plates and sprinkle with parsley.

8 Serve with the sauce and Saffron Barley and Broccoli Risotto.

GL 12 per serving

Marinated Venison with Spiced Pear Chutney

Venison is now readily available in supermarkets and makes a delicious change. You could substitute beef steaks or even duck breasts, if you prefer.

Serves 4

150 ml/¼ pt/⅔ cup red wine
150 ml/¼ pt/⅔ cup apple juice
2.5 ml/½ tsp dried thyme
Salt and freshly ground black pepper
4 small venison steaks, about 2 cm/¾ in thick
1 onion, chopped
2 ripe pears, peeled, cored and cut into medium dice
60 ml/4 tbsp balsamic vinegar
75 ml/5 tbsp water
1 bay leaf
1 clove
1 cinnamon stick
A knob of reduced-fat spread
15 ml/1 tbsp sunflower oil
15 ml/1 tbsp tomato purée (paste)
Sprigs of watercress, for garnishing
To serve:
Celeriac and Potato Mash (see page 124) and mangetout (snow peas)

1 Mix the wine with the apple juice, thyme and a good grinding of pepper. Add the venison, turn over in the liquid and leave to marinate for at least 2 hours.

2 Meanwhile, make the chutney. Put the onion and pears in a small non-stick saucepan. Add the vinegar, water, bay leaf, clove and cinnamon stick. Bring to the boil, reduce the heat, part-cover and simmer for about 10–15 minutes until tender. Remove from the heat. Season with salt and pepper to taste.

3 Drain the venison from the marinade and pat dry. Heat the reduced-fat spread and oil in a frying pan. Add the venison and brown quickly on both sides. Turn down the heat and cook for a further 3 minutes on each side until tender. Remove from the pan and keep warm.

4 Add the marinade and tomato purée to the pan juices. Bring to the boil and boil for 1 minute until slightly thickened. Season to taste.

5 Transfer the venison to warm plates. Spoon the sauce over. Add a spoonful of chutney to one side and garnish with sprigs of watercress.

6 Serve with Celeriac and Potato Mash and mangetout.

GL 9 per serving

Duck Breasts with Fresh Plum Sauce

The Chinese have served plums with duck for centuries: this delicious 'Westernised' version has an exciting, fresh, sweet and sour flavour.

Serves 4

225 g/8 oz/1 cup wild rice
4 duck breasts
2 leeks, sliced
4 ripe red plums, halved, stoned (pitted) and chopped
300 ml/½ pt/1¼ cups chicken stock, made with 1 stock cube
15 ml/1 tbsp soy sauce
10 ml/2 tsp clear honey
Sprigs of fresh coriander (cilantro), for garnishing
To serve:
Minted Peas with Garlic and Lardons (see page 133)

1 Cook the rice according to the packet directions. Drain and keep warm.

2 Meanwhile, heat a large non-stick frying pan (skillet). Add the duck breasts, skin-sides down, and fry for 3–4 minutes until golden and the fat runs. Turn over and quickly brown the other sides, then remove from the pan on to a plate.

3 Drain off all but 30 ml/2 tbsp of the fat from the pan. Add the leeks and cook, stirring, for 3 minutes. Add the plums, stock, soy sauce and honey, then put the duck breasts back on top, skin-sides up. Pour in any juices that remain on the plate. Bring to the boil, turn down the heat, cover and cook gently for 30 minutes.

4 Lift the duck out of the pan and boil the leek and plum mixture rapidly until lightly reduced and thickened. Taste and re-season, if necessary.

5 Spoon the rice on to warm plates. Top with the duck, spoon the sauce over and garnish with coriander.

6 Serve with Minted Peas with Garlic and Lardons.

GL 14 per serving

Fish Dishes

Fish is enjoying a well-deserved revival at present, with a fabulous selection of fish and seafood available at every good supermarket. And no wonder: fish is highly nutritious, simple to cook and delicious to eat. It is also light and easily digestible and contains essential fatty acids, vitamins and minerals that make it a really valuable addition to your repertoire of recipes.

Enjoy it twice a week, if possible – there are plenty of recipes in this section for you to choose something different every time.

Low-GI Battered Cod

Everyone loves fish 'n' chips but if it is cooked in the usual way it has a high GI value. Here's the solution: fish coated in a crisp soya batter and served with celeriac chips and a tangy tartare sauce. For best results, make all the accompaniments first and keep the vegetables warm while cooking the fish.

Serves 4

For the tartare sauce:
2 cornichons, finely chopped
15 ml/1 tbsp pickled capers, finely chopped
1 spring onion (scallion), finely chopped
90 ml/6 tbsp low-calorie mayonnaise
5 ml/1 tsp lemon juice
For the fish:
4 pieces of cod fillet, about 175 g/6 oz each
75 g/3 oz/³⁄₄ cup soya flour
Salt and freshly ground black pepper
1 egg white
150 ml/¹⁄₄ pt/²⁄₃ cup sparkling mineral water
Corn oil, for frying
Wedges of lemon and sprigs of fresh parsley, for garnishing
To serve:
Celeriac Chips (see page 123) and Modern Mushy Peas (see page 130)

1 Mix the tartare sauce ingredients together and chill until ready to serve.

2 Dip the fish in 25 g/1 oz/¹⁄₄ cup of the soya flour, seasoned with a little salt and pepper.

3 Put the rest of the flour in a bowl. Add a good pinch of salt. Whisk the egg white until stiff.

4 Beat the sparkling water into the soya flour, then fold in the egg white.

5 Heat about 2.5 cm/1 in corn oil in a large frying pan.

6 Dip the fish in the batter, then fry for about 3 minutes on each side until crisp and golden brown. Drain on kitchen paper (paper towels).

7 Put the fish on warm plates, garnish with wedges of lemon and sprigs of parsley and serve with Celeriac Chips and Modern Mushy Peas.

GL12 per serving

Crusted Parmesan Halibut with Tomato & Leek Bake

Golden-crusted succulent halibut served on a sweet juicy layer of baked tomatoes and leeks. Halibut is quite expensive, but you can, of course, use any other meaty white fish.

Serves 4

50 g/2 oz/⅓ cup couscous
75 ml/5 tbsp boiling water
50 g/2 oz/½ cup freshly grated Parmesan cheese
5 ml/1 tsp paprika
A knob of reduced-fat spread
2 leeks, sliced
3 ripe beefsteak tomatoes, roughly chopped, hard core discarded
15 ml/1 tbsp tomato purée (paste)
2.5 ml/½ tsp dried basil
2 eggs, beaten
300 ml/½ pt/1¼ cups skimmed or semi-skimmed milk
Salt and freshly ground black pepper
30 ml/2 tbsp soya flour
1 large egg
A little sunflower oil
4 pieces of thick halibut fillet
Sprigs of fresh parsley, for garnishing
To serve:
French (green) beans

1 Preheat the oven at 190°C/375°F/gas 5/fan oven 170°C .

2 Put the couscous in a bowl, stir in the boiling water and leave to stand for 5 minutes. Spread out on a plate and leave for 10 minutes, then stir in the Parmesan and paprika.

Photograph opposite:
Tiger Prawn & Barley Risotto
(page 103)

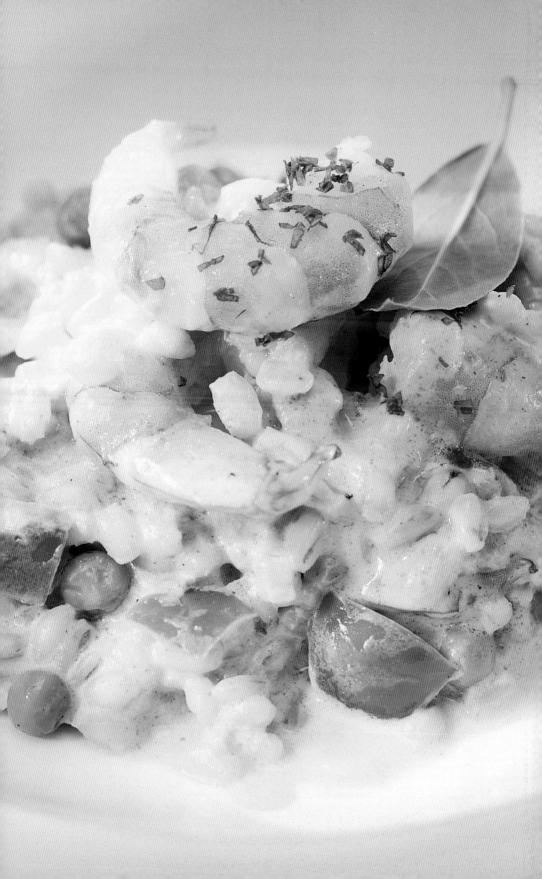

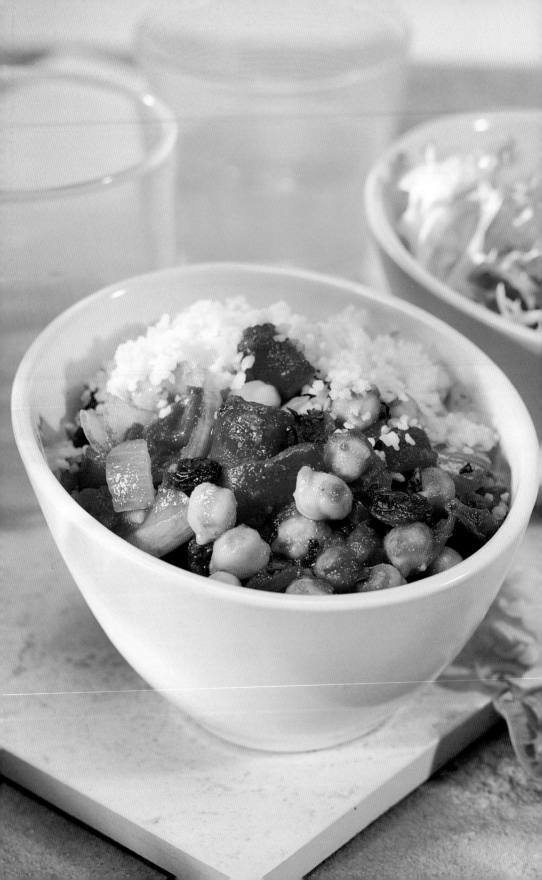

3 Meanwhile, heat the reduced-fat spread in a 1 litre/1¾ pt/4¼ cup flameproof casserole dish (Dutch oven).

4 Add the leeks, tomatoes, tomato purée and basil. Beat the egg and the milk together with a little salt and pepper and pour over the tomato mixture.

5 Put the soya flour on a plate and season with a little salt and pepper. Beat the egg on a separate plate.

6 Dip the fish in the flour, then the egg, then the couscous and Parmesan.

7 Pour just enough oil to cover the base of a baking tin that will hold the fish in a single layer. Put the fish in the tin.

8 Place towards the top of the oven and put the tomato bake below. Bake for 30 minutes until the fish is golden and cooked through and the tomato bake is set.

9 Transfer the fish to warm plates, garnish with sprigs of parsley and serve with the tomato bake and French beans.

GL 6 per serving

Photograph opposite:
Chick Pea & Pimiento Tagine
(pages 112–13)

Grilled Salmon on Wilted Spinach with Prawn Sauce

This is an elegant dish to serve for a special occasion. Cook only the given quantity of potatoes or you'll be tempted to have more!

Serves 4

4 thick salmon steaks
Salt and freshly ground black pepper
450 g/1 lb leaf spinach, thoroughly washed
For the sauce:
A knob of reduced-fat spread, plus a little for greasing
1 shallot or small onion, finely chopped
90 ml/6 tbsp dry white wine
15 ml/1 tbsp Dijon mustard
5 ml/1 tsp clear honey
100 g/4 oz cooked peeled prawns (shrimp), thawed if frozen
Sprigs of fresh flat-leaf parsley and wedges of lemon, for garnishing
To serve:
12 baby new potatoes

1 Season the salmon with pepper and put on buttered foil on the grill (broiler) rack, skin-side up. Cook for 6 minutes on one side only.

2 Put the spinach in a large bowl and pour boiling water over. Stand for 3 minutes until just wilted. Drain thoroughly.

3 Melt the spread in a saucepan. Add the shallot or small onion and cook very gently, stirring, for 2 minutes. Add the wine, mustard and honey and bring to the boil, stirring. Boil for 2 minutes until reduced by half, then stir in the prawns and season to taste.

4 Transfer the spinach to warm plates. Top each with a salmon steak, still skin-side up, and pour the sauce around. Place three baby new potatoes on each plate and serve.

GL 12 per serving

Poached Salmon in Vermouth with Asparagus Bulgar

For a more simple dish, just serve the poached salmon with salad and a couple of baby new potatoes – it will have a similar GI/GL.

Serves 4

225 g/8 oz/2 cups bulgar (cracked wheat)
2.5 ml/½ tsp dried marjoram
4 salmon tail fillets
150 ml/¼ pt/⅔ cup dry vermouth
150 ml/¼ pt/⅔ cup fish stock, made with ½ stock cube
100 g/4 oz thin asparagus tips, cut into short lengths
30 ml/2 tbsp chopped fresh parsley
5 ml/1 tsp lemon juice
15 ml/1 tbsp olive oil
Salt and freshly ground black pepper
150 ml/¼ pt/⅔ cup low-fat crème fraîche
To serve:
A tomato salad

1 Put the bulgar in a saucepan. Cover with boiling water and stir in the marjoram. Leave to stand for 30 minutes.

2 Put the salmon in a saucepan and add the vermouth and stock. Put the asparagus in a single layer in a steamer over the pan. Cover, bring to the boil, turn down the heat and poach for 6 minutes.

3 Add the asparagus to the bulgar with the chopped parsley, lemon juice, olive oil and salt and pepper to taste. Heat through.

4 Lift out the fish and keep warm. Boil the juices until syrupy. Stir in the crème fraîche and season to taste. Do not allow to boil again.

5 Spoon the bulgar on to warm plates. Add the fish and spoon over the sauce. Sprinkle with the parsley.

6 Serve with a tomato salad.

GL 14 per serving

Red Sizzle Mackerel with Hot Soya Bean & Avocado Salsa

Mackerel is high in fish oils, essential for good health. Here it is cooked with lots of spices for added flavour and served with a fragrant salsa.

Serves 4

60 ml/4 tbsp olive oil
2.5 ml/½ tsp cayenne
5 ml/1 tsp paprika
5 ml/1 tsp pimentón
2.5 ml/½ tsp garlic salt
4 mackerel, filleted
1 onion, finely chopped
1 garlic clove, crushed
1 × 425 g/15 oz/large can of soya beans, drained
1 beefsteak tomato, skinned, seeded and chopped
30 ml/2 tbsp chopped fresh coriander (cilantro)
Grated zest and juice of 1 lime
5 ml/1 tsp ground cumin
25 g/1 oz/2 tbsp reduced-fat spread
1 small ripe avocado, peeled and diced
Salt and freshly ground black pepper
Sprigs of fresh coriander and wedges of lime, for garnishing
To serve:
4 medium slices of ciabatta bread

1 Mix 30 ml/2 tbsp of the oil with the cayenne, paprika, pimentón and garlic salt.

2 If the mackerel fillets are still joined in pairs, cut them in half to make eight fillets in all.

3 Spread the spice mixture all over the flesh of the mackerel, cover and leave to marinate while making the salsa.

4 Heat half the remaining oil in a saucepan, add the onion and garlic and cook gently for 3 minutes until softened but not browned.

5 Stir in the beans, tomato, coriander, lime zest and juice and the cumin and simmer for 3 minutes.

6 Melt the reduced-fat spread with the remaining 15 ml/1 tbsp of oil in a large frying pan. Add the mackerel, flesh-side down, and fry for 2 minutes. Carefully turn the fish over and cook for a further 1–2 minutes.

7 Quickly stir the avocado into the salsa and season to taste. Spoon on to warm plates, top with two fish fillets and garnish with sprigs of coriander and lime wedges.

8 Serve straight away with the ciabatta bread.

GL 19 per serving

Fresh Tuna with Harissa & Garlic Butter

It's only the wild rice mix that gives this simple dish any glycaemic loading at all and makes it a thoroughly well-balanced meal.

Serves 4

225 g/8 oz/1 cup wild rice mix
1 vegetable stock cube
50 g/2 oz/¼ cup reduced-fat spread
4 fresh tuna steaks
2 garlic cloves, crushed
30 ml/2 tbsp harissa paste
30 ml/2 tbsp lemon juice
2.5 ml/½ tsp clear honey
30 ml/2 tbsp chopped fresh parsley
Sprigs of fresh parsley and wedges of lemon, for garnishing
To serve:
A large mixed salad

1 Cook the wild rice mix in boiling water, to which the stock cube has been added, for 20 minutes or according to the packet directions. Drain.

2 Meanwhile, melt half the reduced-fat spread in a large non-stick frying pan and fry the fish for 2–3 minutes on each side until golden and still slightly pink in the centre. Remove from the pan and keep warm. Add the remaining spread to the pan with the garlic, harissa, lemon juice, honey and chopped parsley. Cook, stirring, for 30 seconds.

3 Pile the rice on warm plates and put a piece of fish to one side of each pile. Spoon the harissa and garlic butter over, then garnish with sprigs of parsley and wedges of lemon.

4 Serve with a large mixed salad.

GL 18 per serving

Tiger Prawn & Barley Risotto

Barley makes the ideal alternative to rice in many dishes, as it has a much lower GI/GL. Here it's perfect with juicy king prawns. See photograph opposite page 96.

Serves 4

A large knob of reduced-fat spread
15 ml/1 tbsp olive oil
1 bunch of spring onions (scallions), finely chopped
1 garlic clove, crushed
1 red (bell) pepper, finely diced
5 ml/1 tsp ground turmeric
10 ml/2 tsp mild curry powder
200 g/7 oz/1 cup pearl barley
450 ml/³⁄₄ pt/2 cups fish or chicken stock, made with 1 stock cube
1 × 400 g/14 oz/large can of coconut milk
1 bay leaf
100 g/4 oz/1 cup frozen peas
400 g/14 oz raw peeled tiger prawns (jumbo shrimp)
Salt and freshly ground black pepper
30 ml/2 tbsp chopped fresh parsley and wedges of lemon, for garnishing

1 Melt the spread with the oil in a large frying pan. Add the onions, garlic and red pepper and cook, stirring, for 2 minutes until softened but not browned. Add the spices and fry for 30 seconds. Stir in the barley until it is coated in the oil and butter.

2 Stir in the stock and coconut milk and add the bay leaf. Bring to the boil, turn down the heat, cover and simmer for 30 minutes, stirring.

3 Add the peas and prawns and cook for a further 5 minutes, adding a little more water if getting too dry (the mixture should remain very moist). Stir well – the barley and peas should be just tender but still with quite a lot of 'bite', the prawns pink and the mixture creamy.

4 Season to taste and remove the bay leaf. Sprinkle with the parsley before serving, garnished with wedges of lemon.

GL 12 per serving

Tuna Omelette with Fresh Tomato & Basil Sauce

This makes a simple but impressive light lunch or supper. The combination of flavours is superb!

Serves 4

Olive oil, for cooking
1 onion, finely chopped
6 ripe tomatoes
15 ml/1 tbsp tomato purée (paste)
2.5 ml/½ tsp clear honey
Salt and freshly ground black pepper
30 ml/2 tbsp chopped fresh basil
½ bunch of spring onions (scallions), finely chopped
1 × 390 g/14 oz/large can of tuna, drained
90 ml/6 tbsp low-fat crème fraîche
5 ml/1 tsp lemon juice
4 eggs
150 ml/¼ pt/⅔ cup skimmed or semi-skimmed milk
30 ml/2 tbsp chopped fresh parsley
To serve:
Garlic Pitta Fingers (see page 135) and a large green salad

1 Heat 15 ml/1 tbsp of the oil in a saucepan. Add the onion and cook, stirring, for 2 minutes until softened not browned. Add the tomatoes, tomato purée and honey and bring to the boil. Turn down the heat, cover and allow to simmer for about 5 minutes until pulpy. Remove from the heat, season to taste and stir in the basil.

2 Heat 15 ml/1 tbsp of the oil in a separate pan. Add the spring onions and cook, stirring, for 2 minutes until softened. Add the tuna, crème fraîche and lemon juice and season to taste. Heat through.

3 Beat the eggs thoroughly with the milk and a good pinch of salt and pepper. Stir in the parsley.

4 Heat a dash of oil in an omelette pan and pour in a quarter of the egg mixture. Cook gently, lifting the edges and tilting the pan to allow the uncooked egg to run underneath until the underside is golden and the omelette is just set. Spoon a quarter of the tuna mixture on top and fold the omelette over. Slide out on to a warm plate and keep warm. Repeat to make three more filled omelettes.

5 Reheat the tomato sauce. Spoon over the omelettes.

6 Serve with Garlic Pitta Fingers and a large green salad.

GL 10 per serving

Queen Scallops in Pernod with Fennel

Queen scallops are readily available frozen in packs all year round. If your fennel doesn't have many green fronds, use some chopped parsley for garnishing.

Serves 4

225 g/8 oz/1 cup wild rice mix
1 vegetable stock cube
25 g/1 oz/2 tbsp reduced-fat spread
1 head of fennel, chopped, reserving the green fronds
1 onion, finely chopped
1 carrot, finely chopped
200 ml/7 fl oz/scant 1 cup fish stock, made with 1 stock cube
90 ml/6 tbsp Pernod (or other aniseed liqueur)
450 g/1 lb queen scallops, thawed if frozen
150 ml/¼ pt/⅔ cup low-fat crème fraîche
Salt and freshly ground black pepper
To serve:
A large green salad

1 Cook the wild rice mix in boiling water with the vegetable stock cube for 20 minutes or according to the packet directions. Drain well.

2 Meanwhile, heat the reduced-fat spread in a saucepan. Add the fennel, onion and carrot and cook gently, stirring, for 3 minutes until softened but not browned.

3 Add the stock and Pernod and bring to the boil. Reduce the heat to moderate and simmer for 10 minutes until the liquid is reduced by half and the vegetables are tender.

4 Dry the scallops on kitchen paper (paper towels), if necessary, then add to the pan and simmer for 2 minutes only.

5 Stir in the crème fraîche and season to taste.

6 Spoon the rice mix on to warm plates and top with the scallops. Chop the fennel fronds and sprinkle on top. Serve with a green salad.

GL 18 per serving

Pan-stewed Squid with Baby Potatoes, Tomatoes & Olives

This is very Mediterranean. The squid is stewed until tender in a rich, flavoursome sauce of tomatoes, olives and wine.

Serves 4

16 baby new potatoes, scraped and halved
225 g/8 oz thin French (green) beans, trimmed and cut into thirds
450 g/1 lb cleaned baby squid
45 ml/3 tbsp olive oil
1 red onion, chopped
2 garlic cloves, crushed
2 beefsteak tomatoes, skinned and chopped
150 ml/¼ pt/⅔ cup dry white wine
50 g/2 oz/½ cup sliced stoned (pitted) green olives
Salt and freshly ground black pepper
30 ml/2 tbsp chopped fresh parsley
To serve:
A large green salad

1 Boil the potatoes and beans in lightly salted water for 3 minutes until almost tender. Drain.

2 Cut the squid into rings. If the tentacles are supplied, chop them, discarding any hard central core.

3 Heat the oil in a deep frying pan. Add the onion and garlic and cook gently, stirring, for 2 minutes until softened but not browned.

4 Add the potatoes, beans and all the remaining ingredients except the salt, pepper and parsley. Bring to the boil, stirring, then cook gently for 20 minutes until the squid and potatoes are really tender.

5 Lift the squid and vegetables out of the pan with a draining spoon and keep warm. Boil the liquor for several minutes until reduced by half. Return the squid and vegetables to the liquor. Season to taste.

6 Spoon into warm bowls and sprinkle with parsley. Serve with a large green salad.

GL 18 per serving

Warm Smoked Haddock & Quails' Egg Caesar Salad

The remaining anchovies can be stored in a covered container in the fridge for several days. They can also be frozen.

Serves 4

2 slices of white bread, cut into small cubes
15 ml/1 tbsp sunflower oil
350 g/12 oz undyed smoked haddock
8 quails' eggs, scrubbed under cold running water
1 avocado
5 ml/1 tsp lemon juice
1 cos (Romaine) lettuce
For the dressing:
2 anchovies from a can, drained and chopped
2 garlic cloves, crushed
45 ml/3 tbsp olive oil
30 ml/2 tbsp sunflower oil
15 ml/1 tbsp cider vinegar
10 ml/2 tsp Dijon mustard
1 egg
Freshly ground black pepper
30 ml/2 tbsp fresh shavings of Parmesan cheese

1 Fry the cubes of bread in the oil, tossing all the time until golden, then drain on kitchen paper (paper towels).

2 Put the haddock in a pan and cover with water. Bring to the boil, cover the pan, reduce the heat and poach for 5 minutes. Add the quails' eggs after 2 minutes.

3 Lift the eggs out of the pan and put in a bowl of cold water. Drain the fish.

4 Remove the skin from the fish and separate the flesh into large flakes. Shell the quails' eggs and cut into halves.

5 Halve, stone (pit), peel and dice the avocado. Toss in the lemon juice to prevent browning.

6 Cut the lettuce into bite-sized chunks and place in a large bowl with the croûtons.

7 Mash the anchovies with the garlic to form a paste. Whisk in the oils, vinegar and mustard.

8 Put the egg in just enough cold water to cover. Bring to the boil and boil for 1½ minutes only – no longer! Immediately, drain off the boiling water and fill the pan with cold water. Lift out the egg, carefully remove the some of the shell and scoop the egg into the dressing. Whisk thoroughly until completely blended. Add a good grinding of pepper.

9 Pour the dressing over the salad and toss well. Divide between four smaller bowls. Add the haddock and quails' eggs and scatter the Parmesan over.

GL 6 per serving

Vegetarian Main Meals

Vegetarian meals make a lovely change from meat or fish. The recipes I've included here are all designed to be highly nutritious and well-balanced – perfect additions to your GI diet – and will tempt even the most committed meat-eater.

Remember, if you are a serious vegetarian, you must ensure that all the ingredients are brands that are suitable for you. Check labels carefully – everything from cheese to Worcestershire sauce needs to be looked at.

Swiss Aubergine & Sweet Potato Bake

You could make half the quantity and serve it as an accompaniment to Quorn steaks or, if you're not vegetarian, any grilled meat or poultry.

Serves 4

1 large aubergine (eggplant), halved and sliced
2 medium sweet potatoes, peeled and thinly sliced
A knob of reduced-fat spread
1 garlic clove, crushed
100 g/4 oz/1 cup grated Gruyère (Swiss) cheese
Salt and freshly ground black pepper
4 eggs
200 ml/7 fl oz/scant 1 cup low-fat crème fraîche
200 ml/7 fl oz/scant 1 cup skimmed or semi-skimmed milk
To serve:
A large green salad

1 Preheat the oven at 190°C/375°F/gas 5/fan oven 170°C.

2 Cook the aubergine and sweet potatoes in boiling water for 2 minutes. Drain, rinse with cold water and drain again.

3 Use a little of the reduced-fat spread to grease a 1 litre/1¾ pt/4¼ cup shallow ovenproof dish.

4 Layer the aubergine and sweet potato, adding a sprinkling of garlic, some of the grated cheese and a light dusting of salt and pepper between each layer. Finish with the last of the cheese.

5 Whisk the eggs with the crème fraîche and milk and pour over. Dot with the remaining reduced-fat spread.

6 Bake in the oven for about 30 minutes or until set, cooked through and lightly golden on top.

7 Serve with a large green salad.

GL 12 per serving

Chick Pea & Pimiento Tagine

All the familiar Moroccan flavours are here – cumin, cinnamon, sultanas and garlic. A lovely combination, packed with nutrients. Add extra colour by sprinkling the finished dish with fresh coriander.
See photograph opposite page 97.

Serves 4

15 ml/1 tbsp olive oil
1 onion, chopped
1 garlic clove, crushed
5 ml/1 tsp paprika
5 ml/1 tsp ground cumin
5 ml/1 tsp ground cinnamon
2 × 425 g/15 oz/large cans of chick peas (garbanzos)
1 × 400 g/14 oz/large can of chopped tomatoes
150 ml/¼ pt/⅔ cup vegetable stock, made with ½ stock cube
1 × 200 g/7oz/small can of pimientos, drained and diced
25 g/1 oz/3 tbsp sultanas (golden raisins)
2.5 ml/½ tsp dried oregano
Salt and freshly ground black pepper
100 g/4 oz/⅔ cup couscous
300 ml/½ pt/1¼ cups boiling water
To serve:
A large mixed salad

1 Heat the oil in a saucepan. Add the onion and garlic and fry, stirring, for 3 minutes until golden. Add the spices and fry for 30 seconds.

2 Add the chick peas, tomatoes, stock, pimientos, sultanas and oregano. Season to taste. Bring to the boil, reduce the heat and simmer for 10 minutes until the chick peas are bathed in a rich sauce.

3 Meanwhile, put the couscous in a bowl and pour the boiling water over. Stir and leave to stand for 5 minutes until the water is absorbed and the couscous is soft. Fluff up with a fork and season to taste.

4 Spoon the tagine into bowls. Top each with a large spoonful of the couscous and sprinkle with the coriander if using.

5 Serve with a large mixed salad.

GL 20 per serving

Tuscan Beans with Leeks & Artichokes

You can chill this, if you prefer, and serve on a bed of lettuce. It is also delicious with small, lightly cooked florets of cauliflower instead of the artichoke hearts.

Serves 4

15 ml/1 tbsp olive oil
1 onion, roughly chopped
2 leeks, well-washed and roughly chopped
1 garlic clove, crushed
1 × 400 g/14 oz/large can of chopped tomatoes
2 × 425 g/15 oz/large cans of haricot (navy) beans, drained
1 × 410 g/14½ oz/large can of artichoke hearts, quartered
2.5 ml/½ tsp dried oregano
2 sun-dried tomatoes, chopped
Salt and freshly round black pepper
30 ml/2 tbsp sliced stoned (pitted) black olives
Freshly grated Parmesan cheese, for garnishing
To serve:
A large green salad

1 Heat the oil in a saucepan. Add the onion, leeks and garlic and cook, stirring, for 3 minutes until lightly golden.

2 Add all the remaining ingredients. Bring to the boil, reduce the heat and simmer for 5 minutes until rich and thick.

3 Spoon into bowls, sprinkle with Parmesan and serve with salad.

GL 8 per serving

Camembert & Cashew Nut Stir-fry

There is an exciting combination of flavours and textures in this unusual stir-fry. You could substitute unsalted peanuts for the cashews, if you prefer.

Serves 4

2 slabs of Chinese egg noodles
30 ml/2 tbsp sunflower oil
1 onion, halved and sliced
1 garlic clove, crushed
1 green (bell) pepper, cut into thin strips
1 red pepper, cut into thin strips
1 carrot, cut into thin strips
¼ cucumber, cut into thin strips
100 g/4 oz/2 cups beansprouts
1 eating (dessert) apple, cored and chopped
50 g/2 oz/½ cup raw cashew nuts
30 ml/2 tbsp soy sauce
1 × 250 g/9 oz Camembert cheese, cut into cubes

1 Put the noodles in a bowl and cover with plenty of boiling water. Leave to stand for 5 minutes, stirring once or twice. Drain.

2 Heat the sunflower oil in a large frying pan or wok. Add all the prepared vegetables except the beansprouts and stir-fry for 3 minutes.

3 Add all the remaining ingredients except the cheese and stir-fry for 1 minute. Finally, add the cheese and toss until it just begins to melt.

4 Pile the noodles into four warm bowls. Top with the stir-fry and serve straight away.

GL 7 per serving

Creamy Flageolets with Spinach Goulash

This is packed with goodness, delicious and easy to eat – great for a TV supper.

Serves 4

450 g/1 lb spinach
Salt and freshly ground black pepper
15 ml/1 tbsp olive oil
1 onion, chopped
1 green (bell) pepper, diced
15 ml/1 tbsp paprika
1 × 400 g/14 oz/large can of chopped tomatoes
15 ml/1 tbsp tomato purée (paste)
90 ml/6 tbsp low-fat crème fraîche
5 ml/1 tsp clear honey
2 × 410 g/14½ oz/large cans of flageolets, drained and rinsed
15 ml/1 tbsp chopped fresh parsley
To serve:
An avocado and cucumber salad

1 Wash the spinach well and shake off excess water. Place in a pan, season lightly, cover and cook over a moderate heat, without any extra water, for 4 minutes. Drain well, pressing out any remaining moisture and snip with scissors.

2 Wipe out the pan, then add the oil. Fry the onion and pepper for 2 minutes, stirring.

3 Add the paprika, tomatoes and tomato purée and cook, stirring, for 5 minutes.

4 Stir in 60 ml/4 tbsp of the crème fraîche, the honey, spinach and flageolets. Heat through, stirring, then season to taste.

5 Spoon the mixture into warm bowls. Top with a spoonful of the remaining crème fraîche and a sprinkling of parsley.

6 Serve with an avocado and cucumber salad.

GL 13 per serving

Nut & Barley Roast with Chestnut Mushroom Gravy

This delicious roast is very easy to prepare. The well-flavoured mushroom gravy makes the perfect accompaniment and any leftovers are delicious served cold with pickles.

Serves 4

100 g/4 oz/generous ½ cup pearl barley
A knob of reduced-fat spread, plus extra for greasing
1 onion, finely chopped
1 celery stick, finely chopped
1 carrot, finely chopped
1 garlic clove, crushed
5 ml/1 tsp dried mixed herbs
30 ml/2 tbsp chopped fresh parsley
225 g/8 oz/2 cups chopped mixed nuts
100 g/4 oz/1 cup grated Edam cheese
Salt and freshly ground black pepper
60 ml/4 tbsp skimmed or semi-skimmed milk
5 ml/1 tsp Marmite or other yeast extract
2 eggs
For the gravy:
2 knobs of reduced-fat spread
1 small onion, finely chopped
100 g/4 oz chestnut mushrooms, finely chopped
1 bay leaf
150 ml/¼ pt/⅔ cup medium-dry cider
150 ml/¼ pt/⅔ cup vegetable stock, made with 1 stock cube
To serve:
Roasted Golden Roots with Rosemary (see page 126) and broccoli

1 Preheat the oven at 190°C/375°F/gas 5/fan oven 170°C.

2 Boil the pearl barley in plenty of water for 25 minutes or until tender. Drain.

3 Melt a knob of reduced-fat spread in a pan and cook the onion, celery, carrot and garlic for 3 minutes, stirring all the time until lightly golden.

4 Stir in the barley, mixed herbs, parsley, nuts and cheese. Season well with salt and pepper. Mix the milk and Marmite together, then beat in the eggs. Stir into the nut mixture until thoroughly mixed.

5 Line a 900 g/2 lb loaf tin with non-stick baking parchment and turn the mixture into it. Level the surface, then cover in a sheet of greased foil, twisting and folding under the rim to secure.

6 Bake in the oven for 45 minutes, then remove the foil and cook for a further 15 minutes or until firm to the touch. Leave to stand for 5 minutes to firm slightly.

7 Meanwhile, make the gravy. Melt a knob of reduced-fat spread in a small saucepan. Add the finely chopped onion and mushrooms and cook, stirring, for 2 minutes. Add the bay leaf, cider and stock. Bring to the boil, then reduce the heat slightly and simmer for 10 minutes until slightly reduced. Whisk in the remaining knob of reduced-fat spread to thicken slightly. Season to taste and discard the bay leaf.

8 When the roast is cooked, turn out of the tin and cut into thick slices.

9 Serve with the mushroom gravy, Roasted Golden Roots and broccoli.

GL 12 per serving

Baked Ratatouille & Eggs with Dolcelatte Croûtes

If you don't like blue cheese, top the croûtes with Cheddar or even crumbled goats' cheese.

Serves 4

45 ml/3 tbsp olive oil
1 onion, sliced
1 garlic clove, crushed
1 aubergine (eggplant), sliced
2 courgettes (zucchini), sliced
1 green (bell) pepper, sliced
1 red pepper, sliced
½ cucumber, cut into medium slices
2 beefsteak tomatoes, sliced
60 ml/4 tbsp red wine
15 ml/1 tbsp tomato purée (paste)
Salt and freshly ground black pepper
1 bouquet garni sachet
4 eggs
8 thin slices of French bread, about 5 mm/¼ in thick
100 g/4 oz/1 cup crumbled Dolcelatte cheese
30 ml/2 tbsp chopped fresh parsley, for garnishing

1 Preheat the oven at 180°C/350°F/gas 4/fan 160°C.

2   Heat 30 ml/2 tbsp of the oil in a fairly large flameproof casserole (Dutch oven). Add all the vegetables and cook, tossing and stirring, for 2 minutes until they are beginning to soften and all are glistening with the oil.

3 Blend the wine with the tomato purée and stir into the vegetables. Season with salt and pepper and tuck in the bouquet garni.

4 Cover and place in the oven for 1 hour.

5 Remove from the oven and discard the bouquet garni. Make four 'wells' in the vegetables and break an egg into each well. Re-cover and bake for a further 10–15 minutes or until the eggs are cooked to your liking.

6 Meanwhile, brush the slices of bread sparingly with the remaining oil. Toast on both sides until pale golden. Top each with a pile of crumbled cheese, pressing it well down so it stays in place. Grill (broil) until melting.

7 Take the lid off the casserole. Arrange the croûtes round the edge of the ratatouille and serve garnished with chopped parsley.

GL10 per serving

Marinated Tofu, Oyster Mushroom & Vegetable Stir-fry

You can ring the changes with other vegetables but I am particularly fond of this combination of textures, flavours and colours.

Serves 4

45 ml/3 tbsp soy sauce
5 ml/1 tsp grated fresh root ginger
10 ml/2 tsp clear honey
60 ml/4 tbsp sunflower oil
5 ml/1 tsp hot chilli sauce
15 ml/1 tbsp balsamic vinegar
1 block of firm tofu, drained and diced
2 slabs of Chinese egg noodles
1 bunch of spring onions (scallions), cut into short lengths
1 carrot, cut into thin slices
1 small head of broccoli, cut into small florets
100 /4 oz mangetout (snow peas)
100 g/4 oz oyster mushrooms, cut into even-sized pieces

1 Mix the soy sauce with the ginger, honey, 30 ml/2 tbsp of the oil, the chilli sauce and the balsamic vinegar. Add the tofu and toss to coat. Leave to marinate for 30 minutes.

2 Soak the noodles in boiling water for 5 minutes, then drain.

3 Heat half the remaining oil in a large frying pan or wok. Lift the tofu out of the marinade with a draining spoon and pat dry with kitchen paper (paper towels). Add to the pan and stir-fry, turning the cubes for about 4 minutes until golden. Remove from the pan.

4 Heat the remaining oil in the pan. Add all the vegetables and stir-fry for 5 minutes. Return the tofu to the pan with any remaining marinade and toss for 1 minute.

5 Put the noodles in bowls and pile the tofu mixture on top.

GL 6 per serving

Red Thai Vegetable Curry with Sticky Barley

You can use frozen leaf spinach if you prefer. Thaw it and squeeze out any excess moisture before adding it to the curry.

Serves 4

200 g/7 oz/1 cup pearl barley
450 ml/¾ pt/2 cups boiling water
Salt
30 ml/2 tbsp sunflower oil
1 bunch of spring onions (scallions), roughly chopped
30 ml/2 tbsp red Thai curry paste
300 ml/½ pt/1¼ cups vegetable stock, made with 1 stock cube
1 × 400 g/14 oz/large can of coconut milk
1 sweet potato, cut into chunks
1 carrot, sliced
2 courgettes (zucchini), sliced
100 g/4 oz French (green) beans, cut into short lengths
1 × 200 g/7 oz/small can of sweetcorn kernels, drained
2 tomatoes, chopped
100 g/4 oz baby leaf spinach
A few torn coriander (cilantro) leaves, for garnishing

1 Put the pearl barley in a pan. Cover with the water and add a pinch of salt. Bring to the boil, reduce the heat and cook for 40 minutes until the liquid is absorbed and the barley is tender and slightly sticky.

2 Meanwhile, heat the oil in a saucepan. Add the spring onions and fry, stirring, for 1 minute. Stir in the curry paste, stock, coconut milk, sweet potato, carrot, courgettes and beans. Bring to the boil, then reduce the heat to moderate and cook for 20 minutes until the vegetables are tender but still hold their shape. Add the corn, tomatoes and spinach and simmer for 2 minutes. Season to taste.

3 Spoon the barley on to warm plates, top with the curry and scatter a few torn coriander leaves over to serve.

GL 10 per serving

Accompaniments

When time is short, there is nothing wrong with accompanying any meal with some plain cooked vegetables or a salad but sometimes you want something a little more exciting. With very little effort, you can create tasty and interesting dishes that will add extra colour and texture to your meals – and it doesn't have to be difficult either.

All the recipes here are cleverly designed to complement not only the main courses in this book but also any plain cooked meat, fish or poultry.

Celeriac Chips

These are a delicious alternative to potato fries and have such a low GI that they have no GL at all! They're great with everything from grilled steaks to good old fried eggs (although if you're trying to lose weight, I suggest you poach the eggs instead). See photograph opposite page 128.

Serves 4

1 head of celeriac, peeled and cut into thick fingers
Sunflower oil, for frying
Coarse sea salt

1 Cook the celeriac in boiling water for 2 minutes. Drain well.

2 Heat about 2 cm/¾ in oil in a large frying pan. Add the celeriac to the hot oil and cook for about 3 minutes, turning occasionally until golden brown and tender. Drain on kitchen paper (paper towels). Sprinkle with coarse sea salt and serve hot.

GL 0

Celeriac & Potato Mash

When cooking vegetables, always reserve the cooking water to use for stock if you are making gravy or a sauce for a main course – it contains lots of nutrients.

Serves 4

1 head of celeriac, peeled and cut into chunks
1 large potato, peeled and cut into chunks
A knob of reduced-fat spread
30 ml/2 tbsp skimmed or semi-skimmed milk
Salt and freshly ground black pepper

1 Cook the celeriac and potato together in boiling, lightly salted water for about 10 minutes or until really tender.

2 Drain thoroughly, then return the pan to a gentle heat to dry out the vegetables slightly.

3 Remove from the heat, then mash them well and beat in the reduced-fat spread, milk and lots of black pepper.

GL 6 per serving

Indian Spiced Potato, Celeriac & Onion

These are also delicious served as a light lunch, sprinkled with grated cheese.

Serves 4

60 ml/4 tbsp sunflower oil
15 ml/1 tbsp Madras curry powder
10 ml/2 tsp cumin seeds
10 ml/2 tsp black mustard seeds
2 onions, coarsely chopped
1 celeriac, peeled and cut into chunks
1 large potato, cut into chunks
Salt
15 ml/1 tbsp toasted desiccated (shredded) coconut, for garnishing

1 Heat the oil in a heavy-based saucepan. Add the curry powder and seeds and fry, stirring, until the seeds begin to 'pop'.

2 Add the onion and fry for 2 minutes, stirring.

3 Add the celeriac and potato chunks and stir for 1 minute. Sprinkle lightly with salt. Turn down the heat to low, cover and cook very gently for about 20 minutes until tender, stirring gently twice. Taste and re-season, if necessary.

4 Garnish with toasted coconut and serve.

GL 11 per serving

Roasted Golden Roots with Rosemary

These make the perfect alternative to roast potatoes, which have a much higher GI/GL value.

Serves 4

1 sweet potato, cut into chunks
1 celeriac, cut into chunks
1 large carrot, cut into chunks
30 ml/2 tbsp olive oil
2.5 ml/½ tsp onion salt
5 ml/1 tsp chopped fresh rosemary

1 Preheat the oven at 190°C/375°F/gas 5/fan oven 170°C.

2 Toss all the vegetables in the oil, onion salt and rosemary. Place in a roaster bag and seal the end.

3 Place the bag on a baking (cookie) sheet and spread the vegetables out so they are arranged in an even layer.

4 Roast towards the top of the oven at for 1 hour or until golden and tender.

GL 6 per serving

Sesame & Spring Onion Noodles

These are lovely with any oriental-style dish. Sesame oil is expensive and you can leave it out, if you wish – but just a dash adds so much extra nutty flavour, it's well worth it!

Serves 4

2 slabs of Chinese egg noodles
30 ml/2 tbsp sesame seeds
15 ml/1 tbsp sunflower oil
½ bunch of spring onions (scallions), chopped
5 ml/1 tsp sesame oil

1 Put the noodles in a bowl. Cover with boiling water, then leave to stand for 5 minutes, stirring once or twice to loosen. Drain well.

2 Heat a frying pan or wok. Add the sesame seeds and cook until lightly toasted, stirring all the time. Tip out of the pan on to a plate immediately so they don't burn.

3 Heat the oil in the same pan. Add the spring onions and stir-fry for 3 minutes until lightly golden.

4 Add the noodles, sesame seeds and sesame oil. Toss well. Serve hot.

GL 4 per serving

Mixed Salad with Feta & Olives

This also makes a delicious light lunch, served with either plain or garlic pitta fingers (see page 135), which have a GL of 10, or a couple of wheat or rye crispbreads (GL 4 each).

Serves 4

½ small iceberg lettuce, shredded
¼ cucumber, diced
4 tomatoes, diced
1 small red onion, sliced and separated into rings
A handful of black or green olives
50 g/2 oz feta cheese, diced
2.5 ml/½ tsp dried oregano
45 ml/3 tbsp olive oil
15 ml/1 tbsp red wine vinegar
Salt and freshly ground black pepper

1 Spread the shredded lettuce out on one large or four small plates. Scatter the diced cucumber and tomatoes and the onion rings over.

2 Top with the olives and cheese and sprinkle with the oregano.

3 Drizzle with the oil and vinegar and sprinkle with salt and pepper.

GL 0

Photograph opposite:
Celeriac Chips (page 123)
and Cumin Seed Couscous
(page 134)

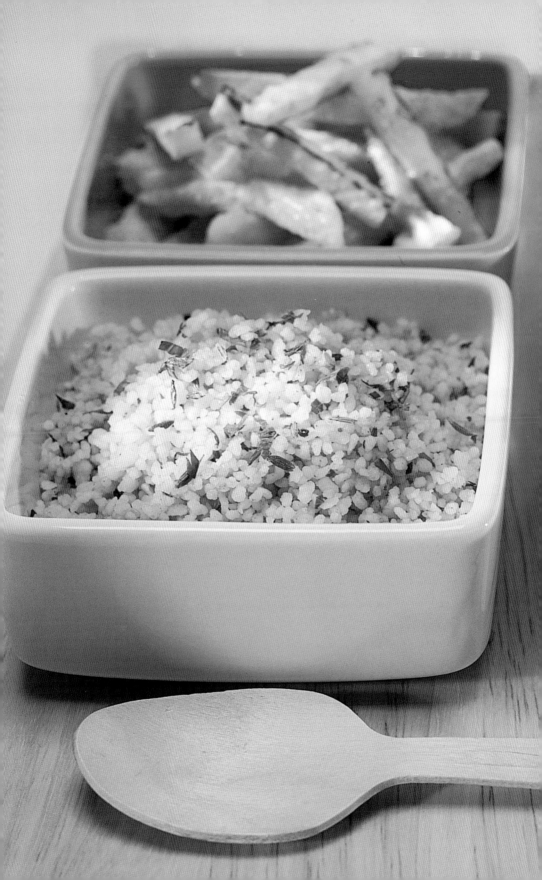

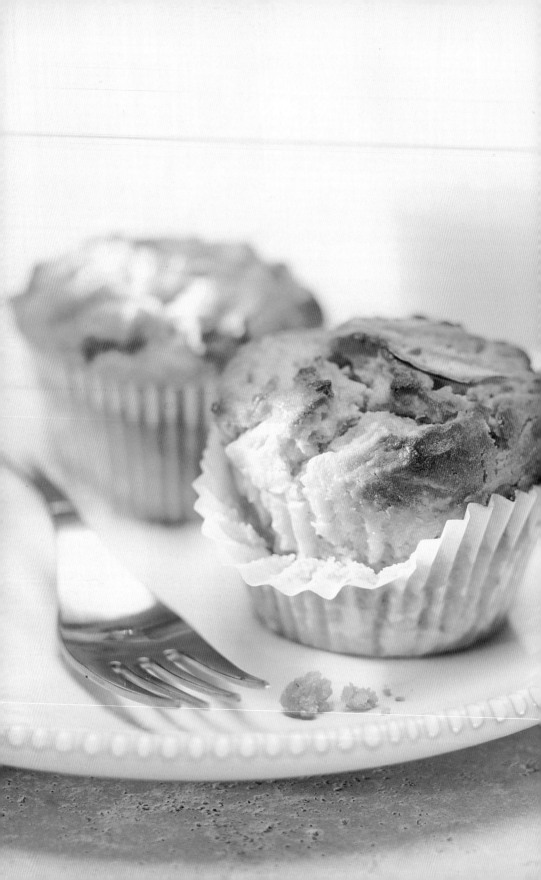

Saffron Barley & Broccoli Risotto

This also makes a delicious vegetarian lunch – try it plain, sprinkled with grated cheese or served topped with a poached egg.

Serves 4

A good pinch of saffron strands
900 ml/1½ pts/ 3¾ cups hot chicken or vegetable stock, made with 1 stock cube
25 g/1 oz/2 tbsp reduced-fat spread
1 large onion, finely chopped
1 garlic clove, crushed
200 g/7oz/1 cup pearl barley
1 bay leaf
Salt and freshly ground black pepper
175 g/6 oz head of broccoli, cut into small florets

1 Sprinkle the saffron into the stock and leave to steep.

2 Melt the reduced-fat spread in a non-stick saucepan. Add the onion and garlic and cook very gently for 4 minutes, stirring until softened but not browned.

3 Add the barley and stir until glistening.

4 Add the stock, bay leaf and a little salt and pepper. Bring to the boil. Reduce the heat to moderate and cook for about 35 minutes, stirring twice.

5 Add the broccoli, stir and cook for a further 5 minutes until the broccoli is tender and the risotto is creamy and the barley tender but still with some bite.

6 Discard the bay leaf, taste and adjust the seasoning to taste before serving.

GL 10 per serving

Photograph opposite:
Honey, Apple & Cinnamon
Muffins (page 153)

Modern Mushy Peas

These are really crushed peas in a light sauce but they taste fabulous.

Serves 4

150 ml/¼ pt/⅔ cup vegetable stock, made with ½ stock cube
350 g/12 oz/3 cups frozen minted garden peas
A knob of reduced-fat spread
Salt and freshly ground black pepper
30 ml/2 tbsp low-fat crème fraîche

1 Bring the stock to the boil. Add the peas and the reduced-fat spread. Bring back to the boil and boil for 5 minutes, stirring occasionally until tender.

2 Crush the peas with a potato masher or fork, season to taste and stir in the crème fraîche.

3 Reheat and serve piping hot.

GL 5 per serving

Crushed Broad Beans with Herbs

If you use fresh broad beans and they are quite large, the skins can be a little tough so you may like to take off them off, once cooked, before crushing them.

Serves 4

450 g/1 lb fresh, shelled or frozen baby broad (fava) beans
Salt and freshly ground black pepper
A knob of reduced-fat spread
30 ml/2 tbsp chopped fresh parsley
15 ml/1 tbsp snipped fresh chives

1 Cook the broad beans in boiling, lightly salted water for about 8 minutes until tender.

2 Drain and crush with the back of a spoon so they are broken up but still chunky.

3 Beat in the reduced-fat spread and the herbs and season with pepper.

GL 5 per serving

Carrot & White Bean Braise

Easy, colourful and extremely nutritious, this is a lovely accompaniment to any meat, chicken or fish dish.

Serves 4

A knob of reduced-fat spread
1 onion, finely chopped
2 large carrots, cut into small dice
200 ml/7 fl oz/scant 1 cup vegetable stock, made with ½ stock cube
1 bouquet garni sachet
1 × 425 g/15 oz/large can of a haricot (navy) beans, drained
Salt and freshly ground black pepper

1 Melt the reduced-fat spread in a saucepan. Add the onion and cook, stirring, for 2 minutes to soften.

2 Stir in the carrots, stock and bouquet garni. Bring to the boil, reduce the heat and cook for about 6 minutes or until the carrots are tender. If necessary, boil rapidly until only about 60 ml/4 tbsp of the liquid remains.

3 Squeeze the bouquet garni against the side of the pan to extract as much flavour as possible, then discard.

4 Stir in the beans and season to taste. Heat through gently, stirring once or twice, for 1–2 minutes until piping hot.

GL 6 per serving

Minted Peas with Garlic & Lardons

This also makes a lovely filling for omelettes for a light lunch or supper.

Serves 4

A knob of reduced-fat spread
50 g/2 oz/½ cup lardons (diced bacon)
1 onion, finely chopped
1 garlic clove, crushed
350 g/12 oz/3 cups frozen peas
Salt and freshly ground black pepper
2.5 ml/½ tsp dried mint
60 ml/4 tbsp water
A few fresh mint leaves (optional)

1 Melt the reduced-fat spread in a saucepan. Add the lardons and onion and cook, stirring, for 3 minutes until lightly golden.

2 Add the garlic, peas, a sprinkling of salt and pepper, the mint and water. Stir well.

3 Turn down the heat, cover the pan and cook for 5 minutes, stirring once or twice until the peas are tender.

4 If necessary, turn up the heat and boil rapidly for a minute to evaporate any remaining liquid before serving garnished with mint leaves, if using.

GL 5 per serving

Cumin Seed Couscous

Cumin seeds marry particularly well with couscous but you could use caraway seeds if you prefer. See photograph opposite page 128.

Serves 4

175 g/6 oz/1 cup couscous
450 ml/³⁄₄ pt/2 cups hot vegetable stock, made with 1 stock cube
15 ml/1 tbsp tomato purée (paste)
15 ml/1 tbsp olive oil
5 ml/1 tsp paprika
15 ml/1 tbsp cumin seeds
15 ml/1 tbsp chopped fresh parsley or coriander (cilantro)

1 Put the couscous in a bowl. Blend the stock with the tomato purée, pour over the couscous, stir well and leave to soak for 5 minutes until the liquid is absorbed.

2 Heat the oil in a small frying pan. Add the paprika and cumin seeds and fry until the seeds begin to 'pop'.

3 Pour over the couscous, mix well. If not serving immediately, stand the bowl over a pan of gently simmering water, cover with a lid or plate and keep warm until ready to serve.

GL 19 per serving

Garlic Pitta Fingers

These are a delicious low-GI-alternative to the more usual garlic baguette.

Serves 4

25 g/1 oz/2 tbsp reduced-fat spread
1 garlic clove, crushed
30 ml/2 tbsp chopped fresh parsley
Salt and freshly ground black pepper
4 pitta breads (white or wholemeal)

1 Mash the reduced-fat spread on a plate and work in the garlic and parsley. Add a pinch of salt and a good grinding of pepper and mix in well.

2 Spread thinly over the surface of the pittas and arrange them on foil on the grill (broiler) rack.

3 Cook under a moderately hot grill until melted, then leave to stand for a few minutes so the melted fat soaks into the bread.

4 Serve cut into fingers.

GL 10 per serving

Desserts

It is very tempting to think, when you are on a GI/GL diet, that you can really go to town with desserts, piling on the chocolate and cream, because you know that it won't add to your daily GI/GL quotas! But, of course, you also know that you won't lose weight or maintain a healthy lifestyle that way.

The delicious recipes that I have put together here provide the solution and give you the best of both worlds: they have a touch of decadence but are also good for you!

Pears with Chocolate Sauce

You could halve the pears and sandwich them together with a scoop of chocolate ice-cream, but you'd have to up the GL by 4, which is a bit excessive!

Serves 4

50 g/2 oz/½ cup plain (semi-sweet) chocolate
25 g/1 oz/2 tbsp reduced-fat spread
60 ml/4 tbsp low-fat double (heavy) cream alternative, such as Elmlea
4 ripe pears

1 Break up the chocolate and place in a small non-stick saucepan with the reduced-fat spread. Heat very gently, stirring, until melted.

2 Remove from the heat and beat in the cream.

3 Peel the pears but leave the stalks on. Stand them in four glass dishes. Reheat the sauce, if necessary, spoon it around the pears and serve.

GL 7 per serving

Apple & Raisin Pie

Using celeriac in the pastry reduces the GI and GL values enormously. Choose sweet fruit so that you don't need to add any extra sugar.

Serves 6

For the pastry (paste):
½ celeriac (about 225 g/8 oz peeled weight), cut into small chunks
200 g/7 oz/1¾ cups soya flour
A pinch of salt
90 ml/6 tbsp sunflower oil
About 30 ml/2 tbsp cold water, to mix
For the filling:
4 green eating (dessert) apples, peeled, cored and sliced
75 g/3 oz/½ cup raisins
Grated zest and juice of ½ lemon
2.5 ml/½ tsp ground cinnamon
A little skimmed or semi-skimmed milk, for glazing
To serve:
Low-fat crème fraîche

1 Preheat the oven at 200°C/400°F/gas 6/fan oven 180°C.

2 Make the pastry. Boil the celeriac in water for about 5 minutes or until really tender. Drain well, then mash. Work in the flour, salt and oil and add just enough water to form a firm dough. Wrap in clingfilm (plastic wrap) and chill for at least 30 minutes.

3 Meanwhile, put the apples, raisins and lemon zest and juice in a saucepan, cover and cook very gently for 5 minutes until tender, stirring once.

4 Cut the pastry in half. Roll out one half and use to line an 18 cm/7 in flan dish (pie pan). Fill with the apple mixture and sprinkle with the cinnamon.

5 Roll out the remaining pastry and use it as a lid. Trim, knock up the edge and flute with the back of a knife. Make a hole in the centre to allow steam to escape and brush with a little milk to glaze.

6 Place the pie on a baking (cookie) sheet and bake in the oven for about 40 minutes until golden.

7 Serve warm with low-fat crème fraîche.

GL 12 per serving

Glazed Grape Custard

This is a low-fat, low-sugar dessert. It's not too rich, so it rounds off a meal perfectly without making you feeling uncomfortably full!

Serves 4

2 eggs
450 ml/¾ pt/2 cups skimmed or semi-skimmed milk
30 ml/2 tbsp clear honey
5 ml/1 tsp vanilla essence (extract)
100 g/4 oz green seedless grapes, halved

1 Preheat the oven at 160°C/325°F/gas 3/fan oven 145°C.

2 Whisk the eggs with the milk, half the honey and the vanilla. Strain into four ramekins (custard cups).

3 Stand the ramekins in a baking tin and add enough hot water to come halfway up the dishes.

4 Bake in the oven for about 35 minutes or until just set. Remove from the tin and leave to cool.

5 Arrange the grapes, cut-sides down, over the surfaces of the custards. Chill thoroughly.

6 When ready to serve, brush the remaining honey over.

GL 8 per serving

Oat Bran Pancakes with Crushed Strawberries

You can also stuff these pancakes with any savoury filling and cover them in a tomato sauce or sprinkle them with grated cheese for a delicious main meal.

Serves 4

For the pancakes:
50 g/2 oz/1 cup oat bran
50 g/2 oz/½ cup wholemeal flour
A pinch of salt
1 egg
175 ml/6 fl oz/¾ cup skimmed or semi-skimmed milk
175 ml/6 fl oz/¾ cup water
30 ml/2 tbsp sunflower oil
For the filling:
225 g/8 oz ripe strawberries, hulled
Finely grated zest of ½ orange
To serve:
100 g/4 oz/½ cup low-fat plain fromage frais

1 Mix the bran and flour with the salt in a bowl. Make a well in the centre and break in the egg. Add the milk and water and half the oil. Beat well to form a thick batter. Leave to stand for 30 minutes.

2 Meanwhile, crush the strawberries in a bowl with a fork. Stir in the orange zest. Chill until ready to serve.

3 Brush an omelette pan with a little of the remaining oil. Pour in about 30–45 ml/2–3 tbsp of batter and swirl to cover the base of the pan. Cook until the top is set and the underside is golden. Flip over and quickly cook the other side. Slide out of the pan on to a plate, cover and keep warm. Make seven more pancakes in this way.

4 When ready to serve, spoon a little strawberry mixture in each pancake. Roll up and place two on each of four warm plates. Top with a good dollop of fromage frais.

GL 10 per serving

Peach & Almond Oat Pudding

This is delicious – try it with canned pears for an equally sumptuous treat.

Serves 4

1 × 410 g/14½ oz/large can of peaches in natural juice, drained,
reserving the juice
50 g/2 oz/½ cup flaked (shredded) almonds
25 g/1 oz/2 tbsp reduced-fat spread
30 ml/2 tbsp clear honey
50 g/2 oz/½ cup ground almonds
50 g/2 oz/½ cup porridge oats
To serve:
Low-fat single (light) cream alternative, such as Elmlea

1 Preheat the oven at 190°C/375°F/gas 5/fan oven 170°C.

2 Put the peaches in a 1 litre/1¾ pt/4¼ cup ovenproof dish. Sprinkle the flaked almonds over.

3 Mash the reduced-fat spread with the honey. Work in the almonds and oats.

4 Spread the mixture over the peaches and bake in the oven for about 45 minutes until golden.

5 Serve with the reserved juice and a dash of low-fat cream.

GL 10 per serving

Individual Summer Puddings

You can use thawed frozen forest fruits if you like:
the GL will be much the same.

Serves 4

350 g/12 oz mixed sliced strawberries and raspberries
30 ml/2 tbsp clear honey
12 very thin slices of soya bread (see page 147)
To serve:
Low-fat crème fraîche

1 Stew the fruits with the honey for 3 minutes, stirring gently, until the juices have run.

2 Dip the bread in the juices, then use to line four ramekins (custard cups). Trim the slices to fit and use the trimmings to fill any gaps. It should use about eight slices. Reserve the remaining slices for the tops.

3 Fill the dishes with the fruit and juice, then top with the remaining bread. Place on a large plate to catch any drips. Put a circle of non-stick baking parchment on top of each, then a saucer. Weigh down with heavy weights or cans of food. Chill overnight.

4 Loosen the edges and turn out on to plates.

5 Serve with low-fat crème fraîche.

GL 6 per serving

Lemon Sabayon

This warm, fluffy dessert has no GL at all. Serve it with a Melting Cookie (see page 150) – GL 4. Try it, too, served with fresh strawberries, remembering to add on an extra GL 2 if you do.

Serves 4

2 eggs
30 ml/2 tbsp concentrated low-calorie lemon squash
Grated zest and juice of ½ lemon
45 ml/3 tbsp Chardonnay or similar white wine

1 Break the eggs into a bowl and whisk in the remaining ingredients.

2 Put the bowl over a pan of simmering water and whisk continuously (I use an electric beater) until thick and foamy.

3 Spoon into wine goblets and serve straight away.

GL 0

Orange Cheese Sherbet

This is cool and refreshing and equally delicious made with a grapefruit, a large lemon or two limes instead of the orange.

Serves 6

1 orange
225 g/8 oz/1 cup cottage cheese
60 ml/4 tbsp clear honey
150 ml/¼ pt/⅔ cup plain low-fat yoghurt
1 egg white

1 Finely grate the zest off half of the orange and thinly pare the remainder. Squeeze the juice of half the orange.

2 Put the cottage cheese in a blender or food processor with the grated zest and juice, the honey, yoghurt and cinnamon. Run the machine until smooth.

3 Turn into a freezer-proof container. Cover with foil and freeze for 2 hours. Whisk with a fork to break up the ice crystals.

4 Whisk the egg white until stiff and fold into the mixture with a metal spoon. Re-wrap and freeze again for about 1½ hours until half-frozen again. Whisk again with a fork and freeze until firm.

5 When ready to serve, spoon into glass serving dishes and sprinkle with the thinly pared orange zest.

GL 1 per serving

Fresh Mango Mousse

This is also lovely made with a ripe papaya instead of the mango.
Make sure the gelatine is thoroughly dissolved or you'll have little bits of
hard jelly in the finished dish.

Serves 4

1 ripe mango
Finely grated zest and juice of 1 lime
150 ml/¼ pt/⅔ cup water
1 sachet of powdered gelatine
30 ml/2 tbsp clear honey
2 eggs, separated
150 ml/¼ pt/⅔ cup low-fat crème fraîche
4 slices of lime and 4 tiny sprigs of fresh mint, for decorating

1 Peel the mango and cut all the flesh off the stone (pit). Place in a saucepan with the lime zest and juice and the water. Bring to the boil, reduce the heat, cover and simmer gently for 5 minutes until pulpy. Remove from the heat.

2 Stir in the gelatine until completely dissolved.

3 Purée in a blender or food processor with the honey and egg yolks. Leave until cold and the consistency of egg white.

4 Whisk the egg whites until stiff. Fold the crème fraîche and then the egg whites into the mixture with a metal spoon.

5 Turn the mixture into four wine goblets. Chill until set, then decorate each with a twist of lime and a tiny sprig of mint.

GL 7 per serving

Bakes & Sundries

Most breads, biscuits (cookies) and cakes have a high GI/GL because they contain large quantities of added sugar and those complex carbohydrates that rapidly raise your blood sugar levels. The problem is that when you are watching your diet, they are often the things that you miss the most, and that tempt you into throwing all your good intentions out of the window.

To help you stay on the straight and narrow, here is a selection of delicious treats that all contain a carefully balanced blend of ingredients. Every one gives you all the delicious taste you want, plus the nourishment you need – and all this without that dreaded surge, then sap, in energy.

Soya Bread

Bread has a fairly high GI/GL but using part soya flour gives a light, spongy, versatile loaf that tastes good but will hardly raise your blood sugar levels at all.

Makes 1 small loaf

50 g/2 oz/½ cup soya flour
50 g/2 oz/½ cup plain (all-purpose) flour
15 ml/1 tbsp baking powder
A good pinch of salt
4 eggs, separated
40 g/1½ oz/3 tbsp reduced-fat spread, melted
45 ml/3 tbsp low-fat crème fraîche

1 Preheat the oven at 180°C/350°F/gas 4/fan oven 160°C.

2 Sift the flours, baking powder and salt together.

3 Beat the egg yolks with the reduced-fat spread and crème fraîche until well blended.

4 Beat into the flour mixture.

5 Whisk the egg whites until stiff. Beat 30 ml/2 tbsp into the flour mixture to slacken it, then fold in the remainder with a metal spoon.

6 Turn into a greased 450 g/1 lb loaf tin (pan), base-lined with non-stick baking parchment and bake in the oven for about 50 minutes or until risen, golden and firm to the touch.

7 Turn out on a wire rack to cool, then store in a polythene bag in the fridge.

GL 3 per slice

Oatcakes

These are delicious for breakfast, as a snack, on their own, or with cheese.
Try having them after a meal, instead of dessert.

Makes 8

75 g/3 oz/³⁄₄ cup medium oatmeal, plus extra for dusting
A good pinch of salt
1.5 ml/¹⁄₄ tsp bicarbonate of soda (baking soda)
15 g/¹⁄₂ oz/1 tbsp reduced-fat spread
60 ml/4 tbsp water
Oil, for greasing

1 Mix the oatmeal with the salt and soda in a bowl.

2 Heat the reduced-fat spread and water together until the fat melts. Pour into the oatmeal and mix with a knife to form a dough.

3 Knead the mixture into a ball, then roll it out as thinly as possible on a surface dusted with oatmeal, to form a round about 25 cm/10 in in diameter (use a dinner plate as a guide).

4 Cut into eight wedges.

5 Brush a large frying pan with oil and heat gently. Add two or three of the oatcakes and cook for 2–3 minutes until firm. Carefully turn them over and cook the other sides.

6 Cool on a wire rack whilst cooking the remainder.

7 When all are completely cold, store in an airtight container.

GL 3 per oatcake

Oat Tortillas

These are lovely as wraps round meat, fish, chicken or cheese and salad. Alternatively, serve them with any main course as a low-GI alternative to bread.

Makes 12

100 g/4 oz/1 cup medium oatmeal
100 g/4 oz/1 cup wholemeal flour
A good pinch of salt
5 ml/1 tsp baking powder
150 ml/¼ pt/⅔ cup hand-hot water

1 Mix the dry ingredients in a bowl.

2 Stir in the hand-hot water to form a soft but not sticky dough. Knead gently on a lightly floured surface.

3 Divide into 12 pieces and roll into balls. Roll out thinly on a floured surface, to form rounds about 18 cm/7 in in diameter.

4 Heat a non-stick frying pan and cook the tortillas one at a time for about 2 minutes on each side until dry and just browning in patches. Wrap in a damp napkin to keep soft.

5 If not eating immediately, store in a plastic bag, tied securely, in the fridge. However, they are best eaten the day they are made.

GL 7 per tortilla

Melting Cookies

These easy-to-eat cookies are very moreish, but don't eat more than one as a snack. They are also delicious served to accompany a dessert.

Makes 14

50 g/2 oz/½ cup plain (all-purpose) flour
50 g/2 oz/½ cup soya flour
2.5 ml/½ tsp baking powder
75 g/3 oz/⅓ cup reduced-fat spread, softened, plus extra for greasing
45 ml/3 tbsp clear honey
5 ml/1 tsp vanilla essence (extract)
20 whole blanched almonds, for decorating

1 Preheat the oven at 180°C/350°F/gas 4/fan oven 160°C.

2 Sift the flours and baking powder together.

3 Mash in the reduced-fat spread, then the honey and vanilla, to form a soft dough.

4 Roll into 20 small balls and place a little apart on a greased baking (cookie) sheet.

5 Press down with a fork to flatten. Press an almond into the top of each.

6 Bake in the oven for 15 minutes until pale golden. Transfer to a wire rack to cool.

GL 3 per cookie

Chocolate-topped Golden Sponge

As this light sponge is not very deep, it can be cut in half and then sandwiched together with 60 ml/4 tbsp of your favourite jam to form an oblong jam-filled cake. Add on GL 2 per serving for the jam.

Serves 9

A little oil, for greasing
2 eggs, separated
75 g/3 oz/¼ cup thick honey
1.5 ml/¼ tsp vanilla essence (extract)
40 g/1½ oz/⅓ cup soya flour
40 g/1½ oz/⅓ cup plain (all-purpose) flour
5 ml/1 tsp baking powder
40 g/1½ oz/3 tbsp reduced-fat spread, melted
50 g/2 oz/½ cup plain (semi-sweet) chocolate, broken into pieces

1 Preheat the oven at 190°C/375°F/gas 5/fan oven 170°C. Grease an 18 cm/7 in square, shallow baking tin.

2 Whisk the egg whites until stiff.

3 Put the egg yolks, honey and vanilla in a bowl. Whisk over a pan of hot water until thick and pale and the whisk leaves a trail when lifted out of the mixture.

4 Sift the flours and baking powder over the surface and trickle in the melted reduced-fat spread. Fold in with a metal spoon.

5 Turn the mixture into the prepared tin. Bake in the oven for about 15 minutes until golden and the centre springs back when lightly pressed. Turn out of the tin and leave to cool.

6 Put the chocolate pieces in a bowl and melt over a pan of hot water or put briefly in the microwave. Spread over the top of the cold cake and leave to set.

7 Cut into nine small squares to serve.

GL 9 per square

Peanut & Oat Flapjacks

These have a much lower GL than any cereal bar or ordinary flapjack. They are also incredibly moreish so make sure you stick to only one as a snack!

Makes 16

100 g/4 oz/½ cup reduced-fat spread, plus extra for greasing
100 g/4 oz/⅓ cup thick honey
30 ml/2 tbsp clear honey
50 g/2 oz/¼ cup crunchy peanut butter
225 g/8 oz/2 cups porridge oats
60 ml/4 tbsp sunflower seeds
50 g/2 oz/½ cup raw peanuts

1 Preheat the oven at 180°C/350°F/gas 4/fan oven 160°C.

2 Melt the reduced-fat spread and both types of honey in a saucepan. Stir in the peanut butter until melted.

3 Work in all the remaining ingredients except the peanuts.

4 Press into a greased 18 cm/7 in square, shallow baking tin. Sprinkle the peanuts on top and press gently into the surface.

5 Bake in the oven for about 30 minutes until lightly golden. Cool slightly, then mark into fingers. Leave until cold before removing from the tin.

GL 8 per finger

Honey, Apple & Cinnamon Muffins

These are as light and moist as any high-GI muffins. Try them for breakfast too! See photograph opposite page 129.

Makes 9

50 g/2 oz/½ cup plain (all-purpose) flour
175 g/6 oz/1½ cups soya flour
A pinch of salt
10 ml/2 tsp baking powder
2.5 ml/½ tsp bicarbonate of soda (baking soda)
2.5 ml/½ tsp ground cinnamon
45 ml/3 tbsp clear honey
100 ml/3½ fl oz/scant ½ cup plain low-fat yoghurt
50 g/2 oz/¼ cup reduced-fat spread, melted
1 eating (dessert) apple, grated
1 egg, beaten

1 Preheat the oven at 180°C/350°F/gas 4/fan oven 160°C. Line nine sections of a tartlet tin (patty pan) with paper cake cases (cupcake papers).

2 Sift the soya flour with the salt, baking powder and bicarbonate of soda into a bowl.

3 Add the remaining ingredients and beat really well.

4 Turn the mixture into the paper cases. Bake in the oven for 25 minutes until risen and golden.

5 Serve warm or cold.

GL 7 per muffin

Moist Fruit Cake

This is a moist and truly delicious fruit cake. Don't be tempted to cut bigger slices though! If you've had a low-GL day, have a piece for dessert with a wedge of well-flavoured Cheddar cheese.

Makes 16 slices

175 g/6 oz/¾ cup reduced-fat spread
75 g/3 oz/¼ cup thick honey
3 large eggs
75 g/3 oz/¾ cup wholemeal flour
175 g/6 oz/1½ cups soya flour
1 eating (dessert) apple, grated, including the skin
250 g/9 oz/1½ cups dried mixed fruit (fruit cake mix)
120 ml/4 fl oz/½ cup apple juice
15 ml/1 tbsp baking powder
5 ml/1 tsp mixed (apple-pie) spice

1 Preheat the oven at 160°C/325°F/gas 3/fan oven 145°C.

2 Beat the reduced-fat spread and honey together until fluffy.

3 Beat in the eggs, one at a time, then mix in the flours. Stir in the apple, mixed fruit, juice and finally the baking powder and mixed spice.

4 Turn the mixture into a greased 20 cm/8 in deep, round cake tin, base-lined with non-stick baking parchment or greased greaseproof (waxed) paper.

5 Bake in the oven for about 1¼ hours or until the top is golden and a skewer inserted in the centre comes out clean.

6 Leave to cool slightly, then turn out on to a wire rack, remove the paper and leave to cool. Store in an airtight container.

GL 10 per slice

Nuts & Bolts

I love these with their added kick of the chilli powder. If you don't like things really spicy, simply omit it. If you find these are a bit of a favourite, make a larger quantity – they keep well in an airtight container.

Serves 6

1 × 425 g/15 oz/large can of chick peas (garbanzos), drained
100 g/4 oz/1 cup whole blanched almonds
5 ml/1 tsp olive oil
15 ml/1 tbsp garam masala
2.5 ml/½ tsp chilli powder
A pinch of salt

1 Preheat the oven at 180°C/350°F/gas 4/fan oven 160°C.

2 Dry the chick peas on kitchen paper (paper towels). Spread them out on a baking (cookie) sheet.

3 Bake in the oven for 30 minutes.

4 Add the nuts, oil, garam masala, chilli powder and salt and toss gently until the chick peas and nuts are coated in the seasoning.

5 Return them to the oven and bake for a further 30 minutes until golden and crunchy. Leave to cool, then store in an airtight container.

GL 2 per serving

Index

Italics indicate recipes